PumpOne®

PILATES

TO STRENGTHEN
& TONE YOUR BODY

DECLAN CONDRON

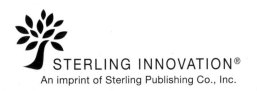

STERLING INNOVATION®
An imprint of Sterling Publishing Co., Inc.

New York / London
www.sterlingpublishing.com

STERLING and the distinctive Sterling logo are registered trademarks of
Sterling Publishing Co., Inc.

Library of Congress Cataloging-in-Publication Data Available

10 9 8 7 6 5 4 3 2 1

Published by Sterling Publishing Co., Inc.
387 Park Avenue South, New York, NY 10016
© 2008 by PumpOne®
Distributed in Canada by Sterling Publishing
c/o Canadian Manda Group, 165 Dufferin Street
Toronto, Ontario, Canada M6K 3H6
Distributed in the United Kingdom by GMC Distribution Services
Castle Place, 166 High Street, Lewes, East Sussex, England BN7 1XU
Distributed in Australia by Capricorn Link (Australia) Pty. Ltd.
P.O. Box 704, Windsor, NSW 2756, Australia

Digital Imaging by Craig Schlossberg
Photography by Susan E. Cohen
Modeling by Kristin McGee
Makeup by Thom Gebhardt

Printed in China
All rights reserved

Sterling ISBN 978-1-4027-5973-4

For information about custom editions, special sales, premium and
corporate purchases, please contact Sterling Special Sales
Department at 800-805-5489 or specialsales@sterlingpublishing.com.

CONTENTS

INTRODUCTION

Joseph Pilates developed his method of exercising during the First World War, initially as a means of staying in shape while interned in a detention camp in England, then as a form of rehabilitation for injured and ill soldiers. With a strong emphasis on muscle strengthening, stretching, and balance, particularly for the core muscles, Pilates quickly became very popular among dancers and gymnasts. Today, interest in this unique form of exercising has spread from professional athletes to stay-at-home moms.

As a child, Joseph Pilates suffered from respiratory diseases that left him weak and unable to engage in strenuous activity. As he got older, he set about designing an exercise regime that would improve not only his physical health, but also his mind. He first developed a series of floor or mat exercises that placed strong attention on balance and flexibility. He incorporated his exercise methods into his training habits with great success and soon became an accomplished boxer, wrestler, and gymnast. Later, he invented numerous types of exercise apparatus that incorporated springs and pulleys to create resistance.

After moving to New York from Germany in 1926, Pilates and his wife Clara (whom he met on the voyage to the United States) started teaching his exercises, which he called collectively "Contrology." Although he trained people from all walks of life, Pilates is renowned for working with the dance community. After his death in 1967, Clara Pilates continued to spread his message to a very dedicated following of teachers and students.

This Pilates book is not just a list of exercises but provides specific, graduated workouts. There are three separate mat workouts, each progressively more challenging. This book will give you the proper form for each exercise as it leads you through the three structured mat workouts.

PILATES PRINCIPLES

Pilates is not just a number of exercises performed in a specific sequence; it is also an exercise philosophy for mind-body enhancement. It includes a number of principles to help you gain the most from your workouts. The six main principles are:

CENTERING

By focusing on the muscles of the torso, you can develop a strong core. Pushing energy from these central muscles to the other extremities can help all muscles function more efficiently. The term given to these central or core muscles is the Pilates Powerhouse.

CONCENTRATION

By really concentrating on what you are doing during each Pilates exercise you can establish that all-important mind-body connection. The more you concentrate on your body as a whole while performing these exercises, the better your body awareness becomes, and in turn, the more benefit you will receive from performing Pilates workouts.

CONTROL

Pilates was established on the principle of control over intensity. It is not just a matter of performing multiple reps and sets of an exercise. It is about how you control your body movements as a whole while you perform the movements. Joseph Pilates did not tolerate sloppy, uncontrolled movements. He was very vigilant, making sure his students performed all movements with complete control. This has become a steadfast teaching.

BREATHING

Deep, controlled breathing patterns accompany each exercise in order to provide the oxygen necessary to move with proper control and good concentration. Full inhalations and exhalations at the appropriate times help activate your muscles and keep you focused.

PRECISION

Proper form and execution is essential when performing Pilates movements. Each movement has a purpose and a place in the sequence. Take time and care to be as precise with the movements as possible for the best results.

FLOW

Body motion should be smooth and flowing, never jerky or sudden. Pilates exercises should be performed with fluidity and grace. This is probably why Pilates became so popular with the dance and gymnastic communities.

BENEFITS OF A PILATES EXERCISE PROGRAM

BETTER MUSCLE SYNERGY

No muscle group works by itself. Muscle groups work together to move your body, and to stabilize and support inert body parts. For example, during Single-Leg Circles (page 20) your abdominal muscles work to help keep your core stable, but they are also working in synergy with your leg muscles to move your leg in a circle. Performing Pilates exercises can help develop better synergy between muscle groups.

BETTER ALIGNMENT

It's very easy to unbalance your body. Whether it's carrying a bag over the same shoulder all the time or using the same motion over and over, we all tend to develop one side of our bodies more than the other side. The resulting postural imbalances can eventually cause debilitating pain if ignored. Pilates exercises emphasize symmetry, balance, and good alignment throughout the whole body.

IMPROVED FLEXIBILITY

Pilates stresses long, flowing, controlled movements. This can have a dramatic effect on flexibility. Pilates movements improve both muscle elasticity and joint range of motion. Increases in muscle length result in better posture and body shape. In turn, increased flexibility leads to gains in strength.

CORE CONDITIONING

The body's core can be defined as the deep abdominal and spinal muscles that support the spine and help to maintain a neutral position. Through Pilates exercises, you can condition your core muscles, making them better able to control movement through the spine. These core muscles are referred to as the powerhouse muscles.

STRESS RELIEF

The controlled breathing and mental concentration required to perform Pilates exercises correctly are great stress relievers. Pilates has been shown to improve circulation, lower blood pressure and heart rate, and decrease anxiety and muscle tension.

VARIETY

Our bodies are very smart machines. When we want to move, the brain figures out the easiest way to do it. Asked to perform a movement again and again, it becomes increasingly easy for our muscles. Changing the task slightly gives our bodies a challenge: to figure out a better way to meet the new requirements. Pilates is a great way to provide change to a workout and give the body new challenges.

HOW THIS BOOK WORKS

This book is organized to provide a progressive exercise plan. It will guide you to certain exercises, in which order to perform them, and when to advance to a new level that will keep you working toward a stronger, fitter body.

The book is divided into three separate workouts. Each workout contains a series of

Pilates exercises organized in a specific order. Workouts can be performed at different intensities by varying the number of repetitions. The book offers two different intensity tracks for each workout: the tone track and the loss track. The tone track concentrates on building strength and defining muscles; the loss track, with more reps, concentrates on weight loss. There is some cross-over between tracks: If you are on the loss track, you will also see increases in muscle strength and definition; on the tone track, you should also see some weight loss.

The three workouts provide an exercise plan, which becomes more difficult as you get fitter. We suggest beginning with workout one and progressing to workout three, even if you are already experienced with Pilates. Workout three can be very challenging, so take your time and enjoy the journey.

Whether you choose the toning or loss track, try to do at least two or three workout sessions per week. Just as the body needs variety, it also needs consistency. Perform each workout for a number of weeks before moving up a level.

A PLAN FOR TOTAL HEALTH

Before you reach for your Pilates mat, take a few minutes to consider the whole picture. Performing Pilates workouts should be part of a plan for total health, a plan that takes dedication and hard work. No one gets fit and strong overnight. Using Pilates is a great way to achieve strength and general fitness, but it is not a cure-all. An overall health plan should incorporate a number of practices and habits that have an impact on your body. There are five essential components to a health plan—strength training; cardiovascular training; flexibility and mobility; a healthy nutrition plan; and adequate rest and recovery. An effective Pilates exercise program depends on all five of these measures. The right emphasis on each component depends on your individual goals.

SAFETY PRECAUTIONS

As with any exercise program, safety is of the utmost importance. The last thing you want to do is to injure yourself while trying to get into better shape and improve your health. When performing these Pilates workouts be sure to pay particular attention to the following:

TALKING TO YOUR DOCTOR

Always consult your doctor before starting a fitness program, especially if you have or have had a chronic medical condition, are taking any medications, or are pregnant.

Immediately stop exercising if you feel pain, faintness, dizziness, or shortness of breath. Wait awhile. You may decide to quit for the day or to resume slowly.

HEAD PLACEMENT

Pay attention to your head placement when performing exercises that require you to lift your head off the mat. If you have neck or back problems, keep your head on the mat until you have developed enough strength to support your head comfortably. Think of your head as an extension of your spine, and try to maintain a neutral spinal position.

NECK AND SPINE

Always pay attention to the position of your neck and the alignment of your spine as you perform these exercises. During rolling exercises, do not roll back onto your neck. Stop at the top of your shoulders. If you have neck issues, you may want to skip the rolling exercises or shorten the distance you roll back.

LEGS AND LOWER BACK

Your legs are a very large portion of your body weight. When they are stretched out on the mat they can put a great deal of strain on your lower back region. Your core muscles need to be strong enough to deal with this strain to prevent injury. You can bend your knees in most straight-leg exercises to help reduce the weight of your legs. Gradually progress to a straight-leg position as you gain more strength and experience.

HEAVY ARMS

When held out, your arms can place stress on your neck and back muscles. Use your arms to help you balance as you learn exercises that stretch out your arms. As you get stronger, begin to use your arms as leverage to increase the difficulty.

FLEXIBILITY

Many Pilates exercises require a certain degree of flexibility; some require a lot. It is important not to force yourself into any position. Never go beyond your limit. If you can not reach a certain point or move into a particular position, modify the exercise to suit your limitations. With practice you will see improvement, and before you know it, you will be performing those exercises with ease.

SUITING UP

Wear appropriate exercise clothing that is neither too baggy nor too tight. Footwear is not necessary and is generally not used, especially if exercises are performed on a mat. A mat provides an excellent non-slip surface for exercising.

FOOD AND DRINK

It's a good idea to eat something at least two hours before exercising and always to have water on hand while you are working out. Right after working out is a great time to replenish the body's energy supplies, while you relax and rest.

TAKING IT EASY

Be sure to follow the exercise progressions in this book. Remember, it is not a race; go at your own pace, taking care not to overdo it. One of the major reasons people drop an exercise program is because they begin too quickly and do not see results as fast as they would like. A new fitness program takes time and patience. It should become a part of your life rather than something you do briefly and then give up.

PILATES PREPARATION

Getting the most out of your Pilates workouts will take some time and practice. There is some amount of preparation that you need to consider before getting started. If you are a beginner or new to Pilates here are a few simple tips to remember:

THE POWERHOUSE

This term refers to the core group of muscles that include the abdominals, obliques, lower back, and glutes. This is your center of strength. It controls the rest of the body. Also be aware of the span of your torso from shoulder to shoulder and hip to hip. Maintaining this box or square is key to proper alignment.

SCOOPING

Throughout this book, you will see the phrase "draw your navel toward your spine." This is called scooping. By drawing your navel to your spine, you tighten all the corset muscles of your midsection, in particular the *transversus abdominis*. Scooping helps to protect your spine and maintain proper alignment while exercising.

EQUIPMENT

Exercises should be performed on a mat, not directly on a hard surface. The surface should be even and clean. For safety reasons, it is advisable to perform your exercises barefoot to avoid slipping.

BREATHING

Be sure to follow the correct breathing patterns for the exercises. Joseph Pilates always taught breathing as a vital part of his exercises. He placed great emphasis on inhaling deeply to fill the lungs and exhaling to the fullest extent, forcing out all the air.

STANCE

The Pilates stance is with the heels touching and toes pointed outward slightly to form a V-shape. Your glutes and core muscles control this stance more than do your feet. Tighten your buttocks and press your inner thighs together to achieve this position.

Maintain this stance when lying down, keeping your feet loose.

VISUALIZATION

Imagery can be very helpful in performing certain Pilates exercises. During rolling exercises, you may imagine that you are holding a small ball in the curve of your stomach. Or during exercises that require you to lie flat, you may imagine that there is weight on your stomach keeping your abdominals tucked in.

WARMING UP AND COOLING DOWN

A warm-up is a crucial part of any exercise program. The importance of a structured warm-up cannot be overstated. It is essential for getting the body ready for activity and helping to prevent injury. Warming up before working out prepares you by increasing the temperatures of both your body's core and other muscles. Increasing muscle temperature helps loosen them, making them more supple and flexible.

Warming up also increases your heart rate and the rate of blood flow to your muscles, increasing the delivery of oxygen and nutrients to them and helping prepare them and other tissues for activity.

A concise warm-up should last 10 to 15 minutes. It should target all areas of the body, starting with gentle activity such as light cardiovascular work, and should gradually increase in intensity, building up to movements similar to the exercises in the workout. The initial 15 exercises in each workout can be considered a warm-up. These exercises start you off slowly and get you ready to perform the more demanding exercises that follow.

Just as important as warming up before exercising is a good cool-down afterwards. Cooling down helps your core temperature return to normal and helps muscles relax and return to their original length. Static stretching during a cool-down can help to increase muscle and joint range of motion, which will improve flexibility and may reduce muscle soreness.

- Lie on your back with your knees bent, your feet flat, and your arms straight by your sides with your palms down.

- Draw your navel toward your spine and inhale deeply as you center your spine.

- Exhale and repeat.

TONE	LOSS
Perform 3 reps	Perform 3 reps

#2 CERVICAL NOD AND CURL

- Lie on your back with your knees bent, your feet flat, and your arms straight by your sides with your palms down.

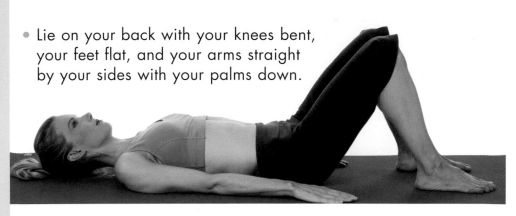

- Lift your head, shoulders, and hands off the mat, pulling your chin to your chest and drawing your navel toward your spine.

TONE	LOSS
Perform 3 reps	Perform 3 reps

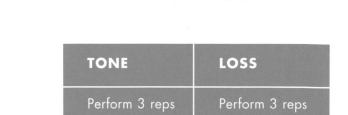

- Lie on your back with your knees bent, your feet flat, and your arms straight by your sides with your palms down.

- Raise one foot off the mat about 12 inches, keeping the same bend at the knee.

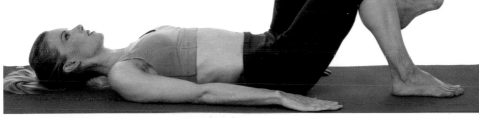

- Lower your foot and repeat with the other foot.

TONE	LOSS
Perform 3 reps on each leg	Perform 6 reps on each leg

#4 ARM CIRCLES

- Lie on your back with your knees bent, your feet flat, and your arms extended overhead with your palms up.

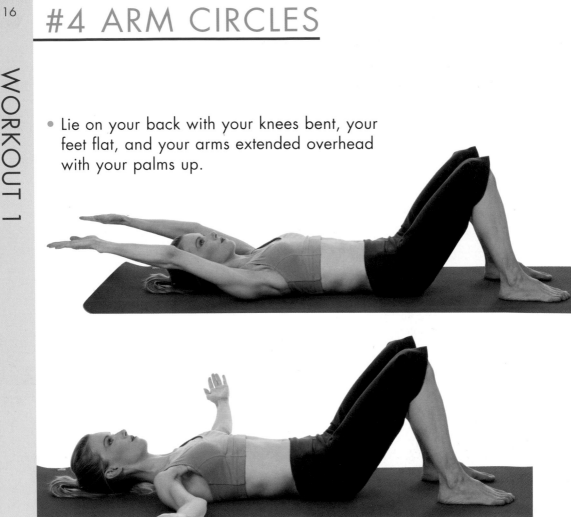

- Rotate your arms, moving them straight out to the sides and then down to your hips, coming together over your body's mid-line with your palms facing down.

- Repeat in the opposite direction.

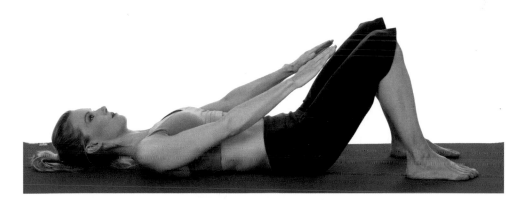

TONE	LOSS
Perform 3 reps in each direction	Perform 6 reps in each direction

#5 BUG

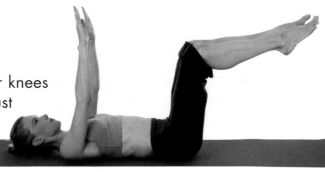

- Lie on your back with your knees bent and your feet lifted just above knee height at a 90-degree angle. Hold your arms straight up over your chest.

- Lower one arm behind your head and also lower the opposite bent leg to tap the mat.

- Lift both your arm and leg back to the mid-position, and repeat with the opposite arm and leg.

- Keep your knees bent throughout the exercise.

TONE	LOSS
Perform 4 reps to each side	Perform 8 reps to each side

- Lie on your back with your knees bent, your feet flat, and your arms straight by your sides with your palms down.

- Lift your head and shoulders off the mat, pulling your chin to your chest.

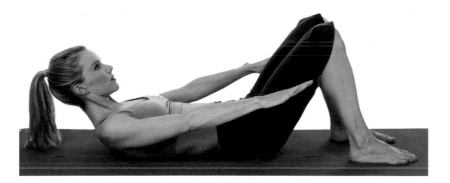

- Draw your navel toward your spine and pump your arms up and down about 12 inches as you breathe in.

- Repeat the pumping motion as you breathe out.

- Keep your head and shoulders up throughout the exercise.

TONE	LOSS
10 breaths with 5 arm pumps on inhale and 5 on exhale	10 breaths with 5 arm pumps on inhale and 5 on exhale

#7 SINGLE-LEG CIRCLES

- Lie on your back with your legs straight out and your arms straight by your sides with your palms down.

- Raise one leg straight up and turn that foot out slightly.

- Rotate your leg across your body, down and around, drawing a circle in the air with your foot.

- Reverse the movement, moving your leg in the opposite direction.

- Repeat with the other leg.

TONE	LOSS
Perform 6 reps on each leg	Perform 8 reps on each leg

- Lie on your back with your legs straight out and your arms extended overhead.

- Raise your arms, then your head, rolling up along your spine.

- Draw your navel in toward your spine as you roll up.

- Continue rolling forward, reaching past your feet. Do not touch your toes; stretch through your arms.

- Keep your shoulders relaxed and use your core muscles to perform the exercise.

- Reverse the movement as you roll back down.

TONE	LOSS
Perform 4 reps	Perform 8 reps

#9 FORWARD SPINE STRETCH

- Sit upright with your legs straight out in front of you and your feet about hip-width apart.

- Extend your arms straight out in front at shoulder height with your palms down.

- Pull your chin toward your chest and draw your navel in toward your spine while reaching forward as if you were rounding yourself over a big ball.

- Reverse the movement, coming back to an upright seated position.

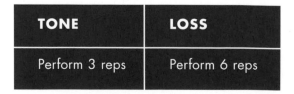

TONE	LOSS
Perform 3 reps	Perform 6 reps

#10 ROLL LIKE A BALL

- Sit upright with your knees bent, your feet flat, and your arms by your sides.

- Lift your feet slightly, bringing your heels toward your buttocks and gripping your ankles.

- Pull your chin to your chest and your navel toward your spine.

- Roll straight backward along your spine until your shoulders touch the mat.

- Roll back up to the starting position, keeping your feet lifted off the mat.

- Hold the same body position throughout the exercise.

TONE	LOSS
Perform 3 reps	Perform 6 reps

WORKOUT 1

#11 SINGLE-LEG STRETCH

- Lie on your back with your legs extended and your arms straight by your sides with your palms down.

- Lift your head and shoulders off the mat, pulling your chin to your chest.

- Bring one knee into your chest, while raising the straight leg to a diagonal.

- Draw your navel toward your spine and draw the bent knee closer to your chest, placing one hand on that ankle and the other on your bent knee.

- Switch legs and hands, keeping your head stable and your back flat.

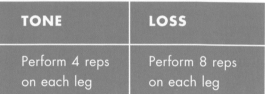

TONE	LOSS
Perform 4 reps on each leg	Perform 8 reps on each leg

#12 DOUBLE-LEG STRETCH

- Lie on your back with your knees bent and both feet lifted to knee height, forming a 90-degree angle.

- Lift your head and shoulders off the mat, pulling your chin to your chest and drawing your navel toward your spine.

- Position your hands at the sides of your shins.

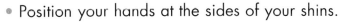

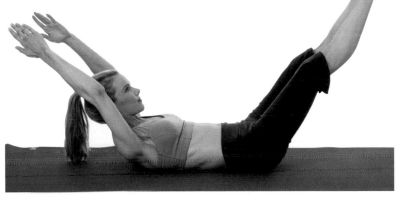

- Stretch your arms overhead close to your ears, and straighten your legs to a 45-degree angle.

- Return to the starting position, moving your arms out to your sides and then back to your shins.

TONE	LOSS
Perform 4 reps of lowering and lifting	Perform 8 reps of lowering and lifting

#13 STRAIGHT-LEG SINGLE-LEG STRETCH

- Lie on your back with your legs extended on the mat, with your arms straight by your sides and your palms down.

- Keeping both legs straight, lift them about 12 inches off the mat.

- Lift your head and shoulders, pulling your chin to your chest.

- Lift one leg straight up toward your head, gripping it with both hands behind your ankle or calf.

TONE	LOSS
Perform 4 reps on each leg	Perform 8 reps on each leg

- Lower your leg and repeat with the other leg, keeping your arms, head, and shoulders up.

#14 BEGINNER STRAIGHT-LEG DOUBLE-LEG STRETCH

- Lie on your back with your legs straight up and your arms by your sides, with your hands under your buttocks.

- Raise your head and shoulders off the mat, pulling your chin to your chest.

- Draw your navel toward your spine.

TONE	LOSS
Perform 4 reps of lowering and lifting	Perform 8 reps of lowering and lifting

- Lower your legs together about halfway down to the mat, and briefly hold the position, being sure to breathe.

- Return to the first position and repeat.

- Focus on using your core muscles to control the speed of your movement.

#15 CRISS CROSS

- Lie on your back with your knees bent and your feet raised to knee height.

- Place your hands at the sides of your head with your elbows wide apart.

- Lift your head and shoulders off the mat, pulling your chin to your chest.

- Extend one leg at a 45-degree angle, then twist your torso to the opposite side, bringing your elbow toward the opposite bent knee.

- Switch sides and legs, keeping your elbows wide apart.

TONE	LOSS
Perform 4 reps to each side	Perform 8 reps to each side

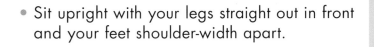

- Sit upright with your legs straight out in front and your feet shoulder-width apart.

- Lift your arms straight up and hold them out to the sides at shoulder height. Draw your navel toward your spine.

- Bending from your hips, twist your torso down to one side and extend your hand to the outside of the opposite ankle.

- Stretch the other arm back while turning your head to look back.

- Pulse three times toward your foot, as if your pinky finger were sawing off your little toe.

- Return to the upright seated position and repeat on the other side.

TONE	LOSS
Perform 2 reps to each side with 3 pulses	Perform 4 reps to each side with 3 pulses

#17 ROLL OVER

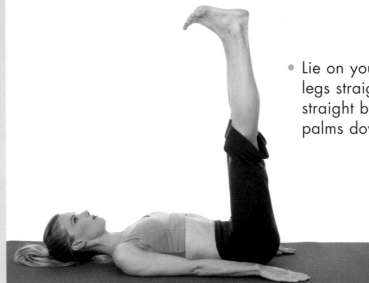

- Lie on your back with your legs straight up and your arms straight by your sides with your palms down.

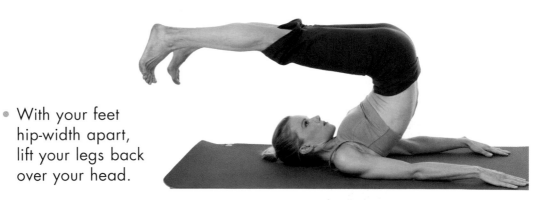

- With your feet hip-width apart, lift your legs back over your head.

- When your legs are parallel to the mat, close your feet and slowly roll back down.

- Open your legs until they are again hip-width apart and repeat for the required reps.

TONE	LOSS
Perform 1 rep with feet open, then 1 rep with feet together	Perform 3 reps with feet open, then 3 reps with feet together

- Repeat the entire sequence, this time starting with your legs closed and then opening them overhead.

#18 BEGINNER TICK-TOCK

- Lie on your back with your knees bent and your feet raised to just above knee height.

- Place your arms straight out to your sides at shoulder height.

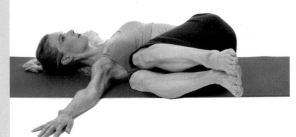

- With your legs together, roll your hips to one side, almost touching your outside knee to the mat.

- Using your core muscles, lift your legs back to the mid-position.

- Roll your hips to the opposite side, again almost touching your knee to the mat.

- Keep your knees bent and your upper body stable throughout the exercise.

TONE	LOSS
Perform 4 reps to each side	Perform 8 reps to each side

- Lie on your back with your legs straight up and your ankles directly over your hips.

- Place your hands by your sides with your palms down.

- Turn your feet out into the Pilates stance, keeping your heels touching.

- Rotate your legs: down to one side, then around and up the other side, drawing a big circle in the air with your feet.

- Reverse the direction of your rotation.

TONE	LOSS
Perform 2 reps in each direction	Perform 4 reps in each direction

#20 HIP BRIDGE

- Lie on your back with your knees bent, your feet flat, and your arms straight by your sides with your palms down.

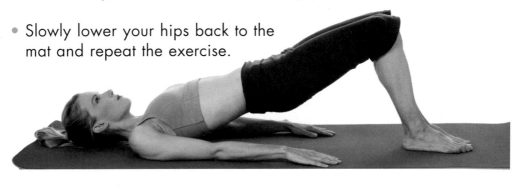

- Lift your hips up off the mat, forming a straight line from your knees to your shoulders.

- Hold briefly, 1 to 2 seconds, at the top position.

- Slowly lower your hips back to the mat and repeat the exercise.

TONE	LOSS
Perform 2 reps	Perform 4 reps

#21 SINGLE-LEG TEASER

- Lie on your back with your knees bent, your feet flat, and your arms extended overhead.

- Lift one leg straight up to a 70-degree angle.

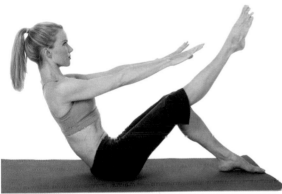

- Lift your arms, then your head and shoulders, to roll up.

- Continue rolling up into a V-shape, reaching toward the toes of your raised leg.

- Lengthen through the sides of your waist, keeping your knees pressed together.

- Roll back down to the mat.

TONE	LOSS
Perform 2 reps on each leg	Perform 4 reps on each leg

#22 BEGINNER TEASER

- Lie on your back with your knees bent, your feet flat, and your arms extended overhead.

- Lift your feet to the same height as your knees.

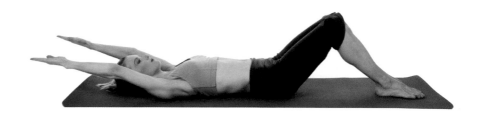

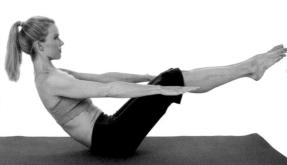

- Raise your arms, then your head and shoulders, rolling your upper body off the mat.

- Continue rolling up into a V-shape, reaching toward your toes.

- Roll back down to the mat.

TONE	LOSS
Perform 2 reps	Perform 4 reps

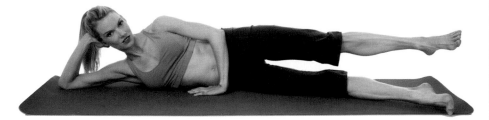

- Lie on one side with your legs straight out. Prop your head up with one hand. Place the other hand on the mat in front of your stomach, bending your arm, for support.

- Turn your top leg out from the hip socket and point your toes.

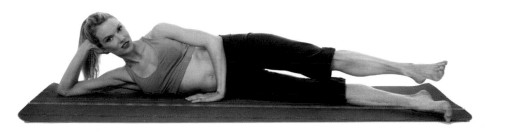

- Rotate your top leg forward to make small circles in the air.

- Reverse the movement, making small circles in the opposite direction.

TONE	LOSS
Perform 4 circles forward, then 4 backward, on each side	Perform 8 circles forward, then 8 backward, on each side

#24 FORWARD AND BACK KICKS

- Lie on one side with your legs out straight and slightly in front of your body. Prop your head up with one hand. Place the other hand on the mat in front of your stomach, bending your arm, for support.

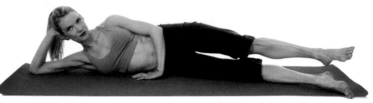

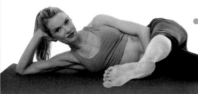

- Draw your navel toward your spine and kick your top leg forward from the hip, pulsing once at the top position.

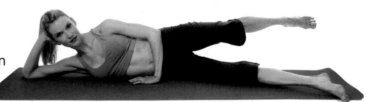

- Swing your top leg back behind and then forward again.

- Keep your hips stacked one on top of the other and keep your feet flexed with your toes pointed.

TONE	LOSS
Perform 2 reps on each leg	Perform 4 reps on each leg

- Lie on one side with your legs out straight and slightly in front of your body. Prop your head up with one hand. Place the other hand on the mat in front of your stomach, bending your arm, for support.

- Draw your navel in toward your spine, and kick your top leg straight forward from the hip.

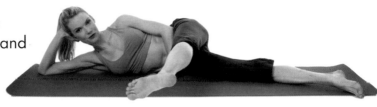

- Bend your top knee and draw your top leg back behind you.

- Straighten your top leg behind, then swing it forward to repeat the pedaling motion.

- Stop and reverse the direction, bending your knee as you come forward and straightening your leg when it's in front.

- Swing your leg back straight and then repeat the exercise.

TONE	LOSS
Perform 2 reps on each leg	Perform 4 reps on each leg

#26 HOT POTATO TAPS

- Lie on one side with your legs straight and stacked. Prop up your head with one hand. Place your other hand on the mat in front of your stomach, bending your arm, for support.

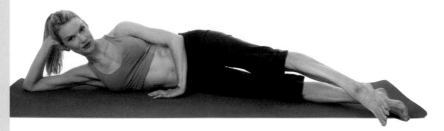

- Raise your top leg slightly, and tap that foot twice on the mat a few inches in front of your bottom foot.

- Lift your leg again, moving it to tap your top foot twice on the mat a few inches behind your bottom foot.

TONE	LOSS
Perform 4 reps in each direction on each leg	Perform 8 reps in each direction on each leg

#27 AROUND THE WORLD

- Lie on one side with your legs straight and stacked and your feet slightly apart. Prop your head up with one hand. Place your other hand on the mat in front of your stomach, bending your arm, for support.

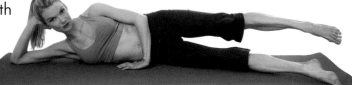

- Lift your top leg straight up, moving your top ankle directly over your hips and turning your foot out.

- Lower your leg, tapping your top foot on the mat a few inches in front of your bottom foot.

- Raise the same leg high again, then lower it to tap the mat a few inches behind your bottom foot.

TONE	LOSS
Perform 4 reps in each direction on each leg	Perform 8 reps in each direction on each leg

#28 BEGINNER FLUTTER KICKS

- Lie on one side with your legs straight out and your feet together, lifted slightly off the mat. Prop your head up with one hand. Place your other hand on the mat in front of your stomach, bending your arm, for support.

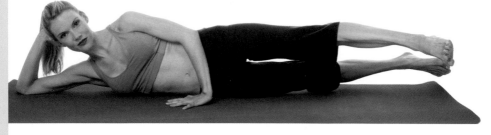

- With both legs straight, kick your bottom leg forward as you move your top leg back.

- Quickly alternate your legs in a kicking motion.

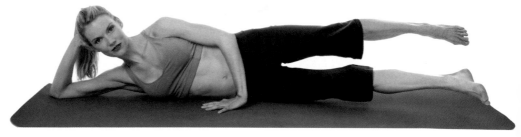

TONE	LOSS
Perform 4 reps back and forth on each side	Perform 8 reps back and forth on each side

- Lie on one side with your knees bent and your legs together in front. Prop your head up with one hand. Place your other hand on the mat in front of your stomach, bending your arm, for support.

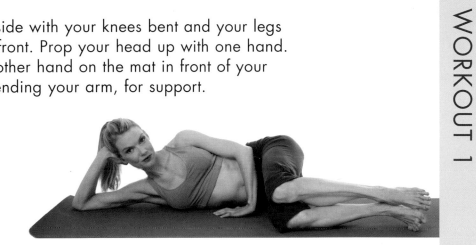

- Lift your top knee, moving from your hip to part your legs while keeping your feet touching and your bottom foot on the mat.

- Do not allow your pelvis to slide back as you lift your knee.

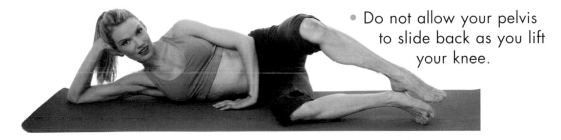

TONE	LOSS
Perform 4 reps on each side	Perform 8 reps on each side

#30 COBRA

- Lie face down on the mat with your legs extended straight behind you, your toes pointed, and the tops of your feet on the mat.

- Place your hands directly below your shoulders with your elbows pointing back.

- Slightly lift your head and shoulders off the mat.

- Push up your chest to a near straight-arm position, pulling your shoulders back and opening your chest. Look straight forward.

TONE	LOSS
Perform 2 reps	Perform 4 reps

#31 SWIMMING

- Lie face down on the mat with your legs extended straight behind you and your arms extended overhead.

- Lift one arm and your opposite leg about 18 inches off the mat.

- Slightly raise your head and upper torso.

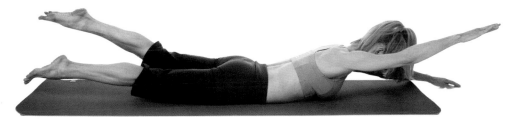

- Lower yourself slowly and repeat with your other arm and leg.

- Keep both your arms and legs straight and your head steady.

- You should feel the whole length of your spine as you perform the exercise.

TONE	LOSS
Perform 4 reps	Perform 8 reps

#32 SWAN

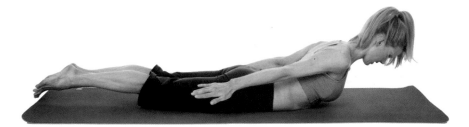

- Lie face down on the mat with your legs extended straight behind you and your arms extended overhead with your palms down.

- Lift your head, shoulders, and lower legs off the mat as you swing your arms into position at your sides, keeping your palms facing down.

- At the top position, only your thighs and stomach should touch the mat.

TONE	LOSS
Perform 2 reps	Perform 4 reps

- Lie face down on the mat, propped up on both forearms with your elbows under your shoulders and your legs extended straight behind you.

- Grip your right fist in your left hand.

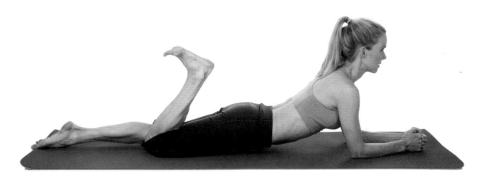

- Pick up one leg to kick your buttocks; pulse twice at the top.

- Lower the first leg as you raise the other leg and perform the kicks and pulses.

TONE	LOSS
Perform 4 reps of 2 beats to each side	Perform 8 reps of 2 beats to each side

#34 MODIFIED PLANK

- Lie face down on the mat with your legs extended straight behind you and your hands at your shoulders with your elbows bent.

- Lift your upper body to a straight-arm position, keeping your lower legs on the mat.

- Keep your back flat throughout the exercise.

TONE	LOSS
Hold for 30 seconds	Hold for 1 minute

#35 CHILD'S POSE

- Position yourself on all fours, then drop your hips down onto the backs of your legs.

- Lower your torso onto your upper thighs and your head to the mat. Move your arms into position along your sides with your palms up.

TONE	LOSS
Hold for 30 seconds	Hold for 1 minute

- Lie on your back with your knees bent, your feet flat, and your arms straight by your sides with your palms down.

- Draw your navel toward your spine and inhale deeply as you center your spine.

- Exhale and repeat.

TONE	LOSS
Perform 3 reps	Perform 3 reps

#2 CERVICAL NOD AND CURL

- Lie on your back with your knees bent, your feet flat, and your arms straight by your sides with your palms down.

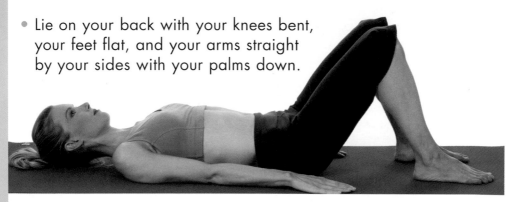

- Lift your head, shoulders, and hands off the mat, pulling your chin to your chest and drawing your navel toward your spine.

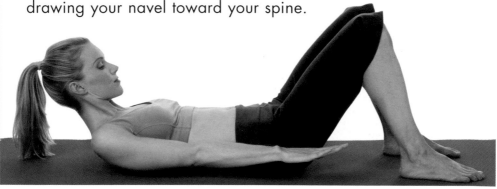

TONE	LOSS
Perform 3 reps	Perform 3 reps

- Lie on your back with your knees bent, your feet flat, and your arms straight by your sides with your palms down.

- Lift one foot off the mat about 12 inches, keeping the same bend at the knees.

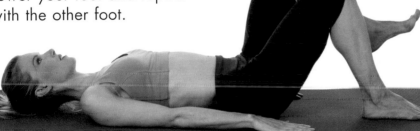

- Lower your foot and repeat with the other foot.

TONE	LOSS
Perform 4 reps on each leg	Perform 8 reps on each leg

#4 ARM CIRCLES

- Lie on your back with your knees bent, your feet flat, and your arms extended overhead with your palms up.

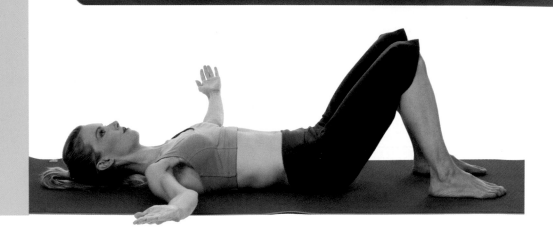

- Rotate your arms, moving them straight out to the sides and then down to your hips, coming together over your body's mid-line with your palms facing down.

- Repeat in the opposite direction.

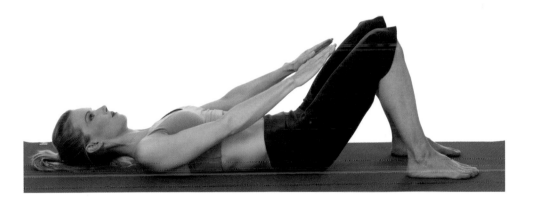

TONE	LOSS
Perform 3 reps in each direction	Perform 6 reps in each direction

#5 BUG

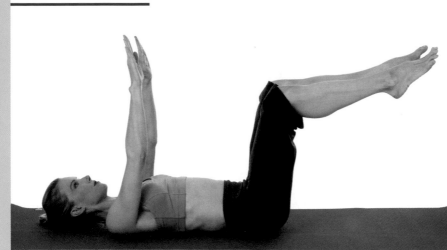

- Lie on your back with your knees bent and your feet lifted just above knee height at a 90-degree angle.

- Hold your arms straight up over your chest.

TONE	LOSS
Perform 4 reps to each side	Perform 8 reps to each side

- Lower one arm behind your head and also lower the opposite bent leg to tap the mat.

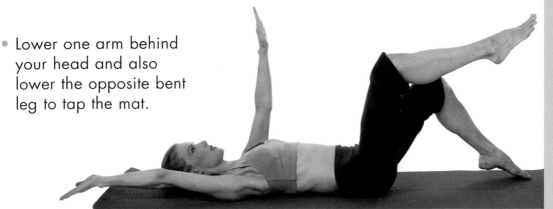

- Lift both your arm and leg back to the mid-position, and repeat with the opposite arm and leg.

- Keep your knees bent throughout the exercise.

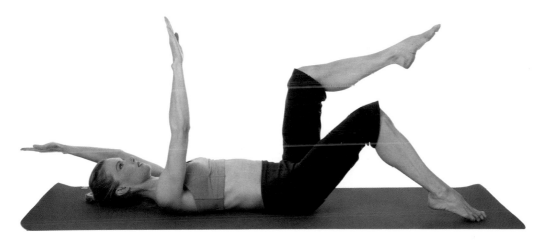

#6 HUNDRED

- Lie on your back with your knees bent, your feet flat, and your arms straight by your sides with your palms down.

- Lift your head and shoulders off the mat, pulling your chin to your chest.

- Bring your feet up to knee level.

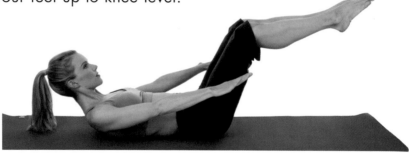

- Draw your navel toward your spine and pump your arms up and down about 12 inches as you breathe in.

- Repeat the pumping motion as you breathe out.

- Keep your head and shoulders up throughout the exercise.

TONE	LOSS
10 breaths with 5 arm pumps on inhale and 5 on exhale	10 breaths with 5 arm pumps on inhale and 5 on exhale

#7 SINGLE-LEG CIRCLES

- Lie on your back with your legs straight out and your arms straight by your sides with your palms down.

- Raise one leg straight up and turn that foot out slightly.

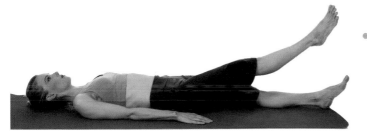

- Rotate your leg across your body, down and around, drawing a circle in the air with your foot.

- Reverse the movement, moving your leg in the opposite direction.

- Repeat with the other leg.

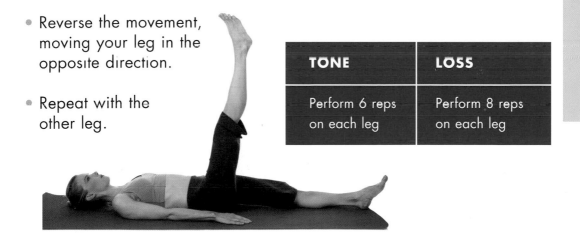

TONE	LOSS
Perform 6 reps on each leg	Perform 8 reps on each leg

#8 ROLL UP

- Lie on your back with your legs straight out and your arms extended overhead.

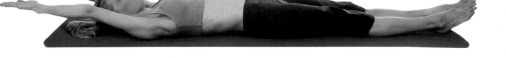

- Raise your arms, then your head, rolling up along your spine.

- Draw your navel in toward your spine as you roll up.

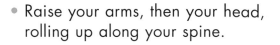

- Continue rolling forward, reaching past your feet. Do not touch your toes; stretch through your arms.

- Keep your shoulders relaxed and use your core muscles to perform the exercise.

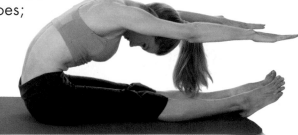

- Reverse the movement as you roll back down.

TONE	LOSS
Perform 4 reps	Perform 8 reps

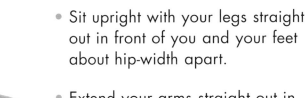

- Sit upright with your legs straight out in front of you and your feet about hip-width apart.

- Extend your arms straight out in front at shoulder height with your palms down.

- Pull your chin toward your chest and draw your navel in toward your spine while reaching forward as if you were rounding yourself over a big ball.

- Reverse the movement, coming back to an upright seated position.

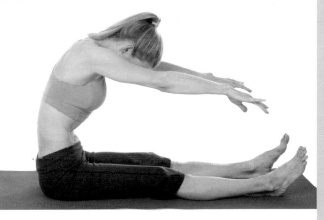

TONE	LOSS
Perform 3 reps	Perform 6 reps

#10 ROLL LIKE A BALL

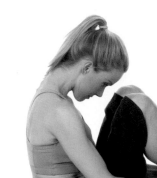

- Sit upright with your knees bent, your feet flat, and your arms by your sides.

- Lift your feet slightly, bringing your heels toward your buttocks and gripping your ankles.

- Pull your chin to your chest and your navel toward your spine.

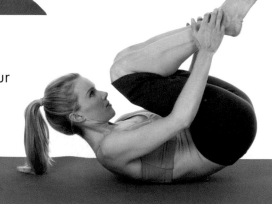

- Roll straight backward along your spine until your shoulders touch the mat.

- Roll back up to the starting position, keeping your feet lifted off the mat.

- Hold the same body position throughout the exercise.

TONE	LOSS
Perform 3 reps	Perform 6 reps

#11 SINGLE-LEG STRETCH

- Lie on your back with your legs extended and your arms straight by your sides with your palms down.

- Lift your head and shoulders off the mat, pulling your chin to your chest.

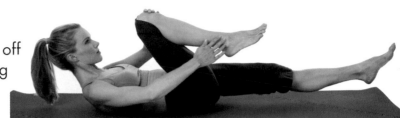

- Bring one knee into your chest, while slightly raising the straight leg to a diagonal.

- Draw your navel toward your spine and draw the bent knee closer to your chest, placing one hand on your ankle and the other on your bent knee.

- Switch legs and hands, keeping your head stable and your back flat.

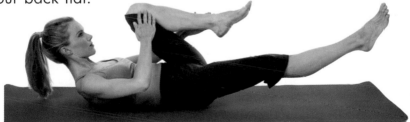

TONE	LOSS
Perform 4 reps on each leg	Perform 8 reps on each leg

#12 DOUBLE-LEG STRETCH

- Lie on your back with your knees bent and both feet lifted to knee height, forming a 90-degree angle.

- Lift your head and shoulders off the mat, pulling your chin to your chest, and drawing your navel toward your spine.

- Position your hands at the sides of your shins.

- Stretch your arms overhead close to your ears, and straighten your legs to a 45-degree angle.

- Return to the starting position, moving your arms out to your sides, and then back to your shins.

TONE	LOSS
Perform 4 reps of lowering and lifting	Perform 8 reps of lowering and lifting

#13 STRAIGHT-LEG SINGLE-LEG STRETCH

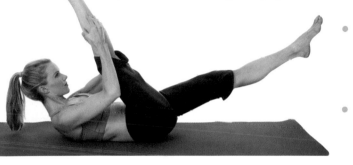

- Lie on your back with your legs extended on the mat, with your arms straight by your sides and your palms down.

- Keeping both legs straight, lift them about 12 inches off the mat.

- Lift your head and shoulders, pulling your chin to your chest.

- Lift one leg straight up toward your head, gripping it with both hands behind your ankle or calf.

- Lower your leg and repeat with the other leg, keeping your arms, head, and shoulders up.

TONE	LOSS
Perform 4 reps on each leg	Perform 8 reps on each leg

#14 STRAIGHT-LEG DOUBLE-LEG STRETCH

- Lie on your back with your legs straight up and your hands at the sides of your head.

- Raise your head and shoulders off the mat, pulling your chin to your chest.

- Draw your navel toward your spine.

TONE	LOSS
Perform 4 reps of lowering and lifting	Perform 8 reps of lowering and lifting

- Lower your legs together about halfway down to the mat, and briefly hold the position, being sure to breathe.

- Return to the first position and repeat.

- Focus on using your core muscles to control the speed of your movement.

#15 CRISS CROSS

- Lie on your back with your knees bent and your feet raised to knee height.

- Place your hands at the sides of your head with your elbows wide apart.

- Lift your head and shoulders off the mat, pulling your chin to your chest.

- Extend one leg at a 45-degree angle, then twist your torso to the opposite side, bringing your elbow toward the opposite bent knee.

- Switch sides and legs, keeping your elbows wide apart.

TONE	LOSS
Perform 4 reps to each side	Perform 8 reps to each side

#16 SAW

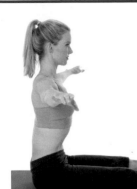

- Sit upright with your legs straight out in front and your feet shoulder-width apart.

- Lift your arms straight up and hold them out to the sides at shoulder height. Draw your navel toward your spine.

- Bending from your hips, twist your torso down to one side and extend your hand to the outside of the opposite ankle.

- Stretch the other arm back while turning your head to look back.

- Pulse three times toward your foot, as if your pinky finger were sawing off your little toe.

- Return to the upright seated position and repeat on the other side.

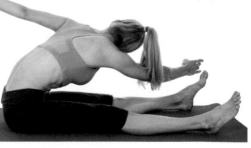

TONE	LOSS
Perform 2 reps to each side with 3 pulses	Perform 4 reps to each side with 3 pulses

#17 OPEN-LEG ROCKER

- Sit with your knees bent, your feet flat, and your hands on your ankles.

- Draw your navel in toward your spine.

- Sit back on your buttocks and lift your feet off the mat, bringing them up to knee height.

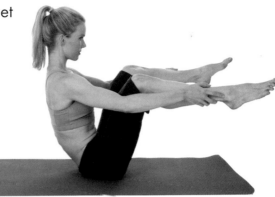

- Separate your feet to about shoulder width and roll back onto the top of your back.

- Roll back to the upright position.

- Keep your legs bent and your feet apart throughout the exercise.

TONE	LOSS
Perform 3 reps	Perform 6 reps

#18 ROLL OVER

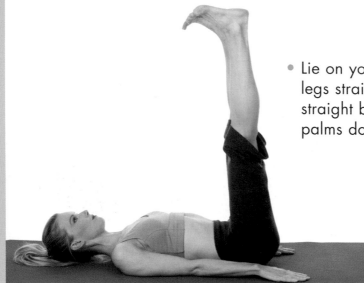

- Lie on your back with your legs straight up and your arms straight by your sides with your palms down.

- With your feet hip-width apart, lift your legs back over your head.

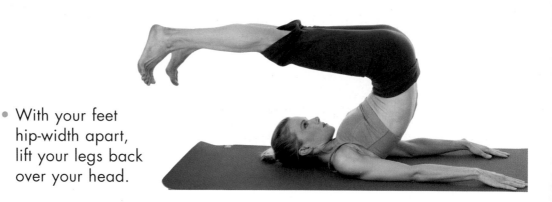

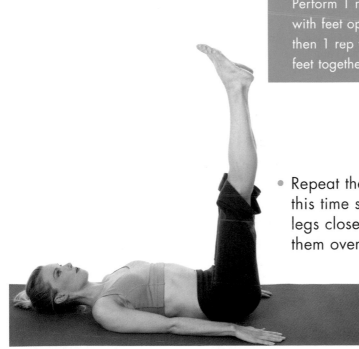

- When your legs are parallel to the mat, close your feet and slowly roll back down.

- Open your legs until they are again hip-width apart and repeat for the required reps.

TONE	LOSS
Perform 1 rep with feet open, then 1 rep with feet together	Perform 3 reps with feet open, then 3 reps with feet together

- Repeat the entire sequence, this time starting with your legs closed and then opening them overhead.

#19 TICK TOCK

- Lie on your back with your legs straight up and your ankles directly over your hips.

- Position your arms straight out to your sides at shoulder height.

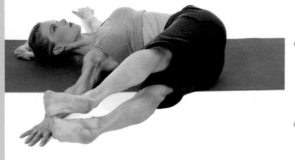

- With your legs together, roll your hips to one side, almost touching your outside foot to the mat.

- Using your core muscles, lift your legs back to the mid-position.

- Roll your hips to the opposite side, again almost touching your foot to the mat.

- Keep your legs straight and your upper body stable throughout.

TONE	LOSS
Perform 4 reps to each side	Perform 8 reps to each side

- Lie on your back with your legs straight up and your ankles directly over your hips.

- Place your hands by your sides with your palms down.

- Turn your feet out into the Pilates stance, keeping your heels touching.

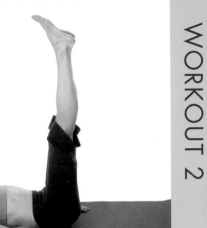

- Rotate your legs: down to one side, then around and up the other side, drawing a big circle in the air with your feet.

- Reverse the direction of your rotation.

TONE	LOSS
Perform 4 reps in each direction	Perform 8 reps in each direction

#21 ADVANCED CORKSCREW

- Lie on your back with your legs straight up at a 45-degree angle.

- Place your hands by your sides with your palms down.

- Turn your feet out into the Pilates stance, keeping your heels touching.

- Roll back to lower your legs behind your head, rolling onto your shoulders.

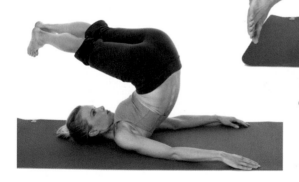

- Using your core muscles, rotate your legs around your head and down at a 45-degree angle, drawing a big circle in the air.

- Reverse the direction of your rotation.

TONE	LOSS
Perform 2 reps in each direction	Perform 4 reps in each direction

- Lie on your back with your knees bent, your feet flat, and your arms straight by your sides with your palms down.

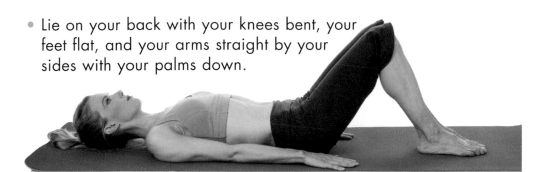

- Lift your hips off the mat, forming a straight line from your knees to your shoulders.

- Hold briefly, 1 to 2 seconds, at the top position.

- Slowly lower your hips back to the mat and repeat the exercise.

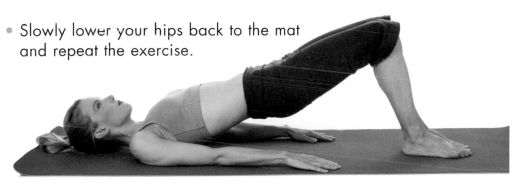

TONE	LOSS
Perform 2 reps	Perform 4 reps

#23 EXTENDED-LEG HIP BRIDGE

- Lie on your back with your knees bent, your feet flat, and your arms straight by your sides with your palms down.

- Lift your hips off the mat, forming a straight line from your knees to your shoulders.

- Extend one leg straight out and point your foot.

- Lower yourself back to the mat and repeat the exercise with your other leg.

TONE	LOSS
Perform 4 reps on each leg	Perform 8 reps on each leg

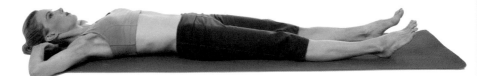

- Lie on your back with your legs extended and your feet hip-width apart.

- Position your hands at the sides of your head with your elbows out to the sides.

- Carefully roll up off the mat, pulling your navel in toward your spine.

- Continue rolling forward toward your feet, lowering your head to your knees.

- Sit up straight and start to lean back at an angle, then reverse the movement, rolling back to the starting position.

- Keep your elbows wide throughout the exercise.

TONE	LOSS
Perform 2 reps	Perform 4 reps

#25 SHAVING

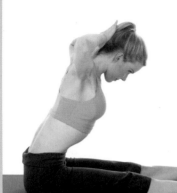

- Sit upright with your legs extended straight out in front and your feet hip-width apart.

- Position your hands behind your head with your elbows out to the sides. Lean slightly forward from your hips and hold your thumb and index fingers together.

- Straighten your arms overhead at a 45-degree angle, as if you were shaving the back of your neck.

- Move your hands back behind your head and repeat the exercise.

- Keep your back flat throughout the exercise and be sure your palms face your head. Relax your shoulders as you stretch your arms out and back.

TONE	LOSS
Perform 8 reps	Perform 16 reps

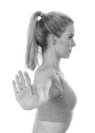

- Sit upright with your legs extended straight out in front and your feet shoulder-width apart.

- Lift your arms straight up and out to the sides at shoulder height with your hands pointing up.

- Draw your navel toward your spine and twist from your waist 90 degrees to one side.

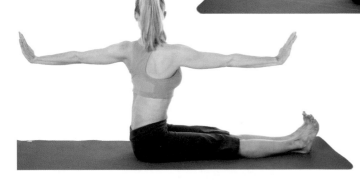

- Twist back to the middle, and then to the opposite side.

- Keep your arms up at shoulder height and your fingers pointing up throughout the exercise.

TONE	LOSS
Perform 2 reps to each side	Perform 4 reps to each side

#27 INCLINE PLANK

WORKOUT 2

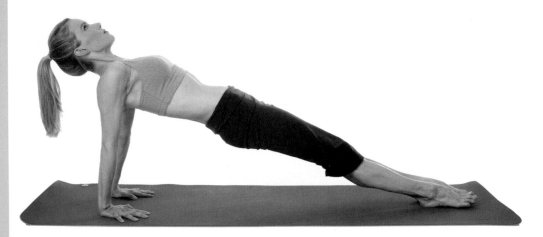

- Sit on the mat with your legs extended straight out in front.

- Position your hands about 12 inches behind your buttocks with your palms down.

- Lift your hips off the mat, keeping your legs straight and your feet pointed.

- Come up into a straight-arm position and hold it briefly.

- Keep your head up and look toward the ceiling.

TONE	LOSS
Hold for 30 seconds	Hold for 1 minute

- Lie flat on your back with your knees bent, your feet flat, and your arms extended overhead.

- Lift one leg straight up to a 70-degree angle.

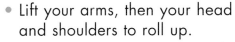

- Lift your arms, then your head and shoulders to roll up.

- Continue rolling up into a V-shape, reaching toward the toes of your raised leg.

- Lengthen through the sides of your waist, keeping your knees pressed together.

- Roll back down to the mat.

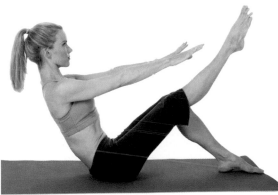

TONE	LOSS
Perform 2 reps on each leg	Perform 4 reps on each leg

#29 SINGLE-LEG TEASER WITH TWIST

- Lie flat on your back with your knees bent, your feet flat, and your arms extended overhead.

- Lift one leg straight up to a 70-degree angle.

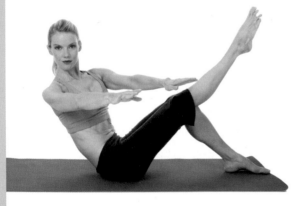

- Lift your arms, then your head and shoulders, to roll up.

- Continue rolling up into a V-shape, reaching toward the toes of your raised leg.

- Twist your torso, shoulders, and head to the raised-leg side.

- Lengthen through the sides of your waist, keeping your knees pressed together.

- Straighten your torso and roll back down to the mat.

TONE	LOSS
Perform 2 reps on each leg	Perform 4 reps on each leg

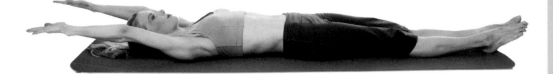

- Lie flat on your back with your arms extended overhead and your legs straight out in front.

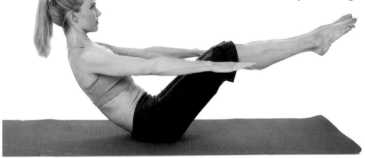

- Lift your legs to a 45-degree angle with your knees bent.

- Raise your arms, then your head and shoulders, to roll up.

- Continue rolling up into a V-shape, reaching toward your toes.

- Roll back down to the mat.

TONE	LOSS
Perform 2 reps	Perform 4 reps

#31 TEASER WITH TWIST

- Lie flat on your back with your arms extended overhead and your legs straight out in front.

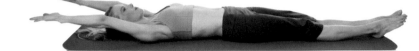

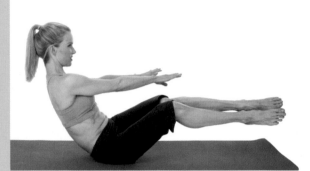

- Raise your legs to a 45-degree angle with your knees bent.

- Raise your arms, then your head and shoulders, rolling your upper body off the mat.

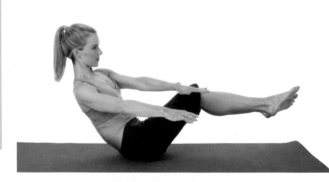

- Continue rolling up into a V-shape, reaching toward your toes.

- Twist your torso, shoulders, and head to one side.

- Straighten your torso and roll back down to the mat.

TONE	LOSS
Perform 2 reps to each side	Perform 4 reps to each side

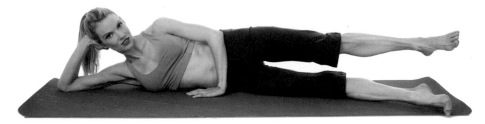

- Lie on one side with your legs straight out. Prop up your head with one hand. Place the other hand on the mat in front of your stomach, bending your arm, for support.

- Turn your top leg out from the hip socket and point your toes.

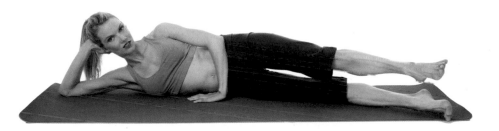

- Rotate your top leg forward, to make small circles in the air.

- Reverse the movement, making small circles in the opposite direction.

TONE	LOSS
Perform 4 circles forward, then 4 backward, on each side	Perform 8 circles forward, then 8 backward, on each side

#33 FORWARD AND BACK KICKS

- Lie on one side with your legs out straight and slightly in front of your body. Prop your head up with one hand. Place the other hand on the mat in front of your stomach, bending your arm, for support.

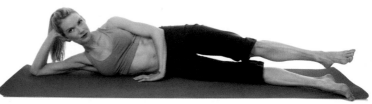

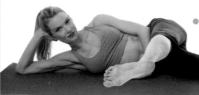

- Draw your navel toward your spine and kick your top leg forward from the hip, pulsing once at the top position.

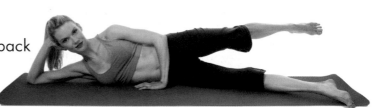

- Swing your top leg back behind and then forward again.

- Keep your hips stacked one on top of the other and keep your feet flexed with your toes pointed.

TONE	LOSS
Perform 4 reps on each leg	Perform 8 reps on each leg

- Lie on one side with your legs out straight and slightly in front of your body. Prop your head up with one hand. Place the other hand on the mat in front of your stomach, bending your arm, for support.

- Draw your navel in toward your spine and kick your top leg forward from the hip.

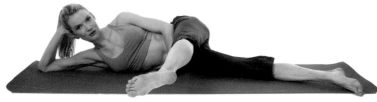

- Bend your top knee and draw your top leg back behind you.

- Straighten your top leg behind, then swing it forward to repeat the pedaling motion.

- Stop and reverse the direction, bending your knee as you come forward and straightening your leg when it's in front.

- Swing your leg back straight and then repeat the exercise.

TONE	LOSS
Perform 2 reps on each leg	Perform 4 reps on each leg

#35 HOT POTATO TAPS

- Lie on one side with your legs straight and stacked. Prop up your head with one hand. Place your other hand on the mat in front of your stomach, bending your arm, for support.

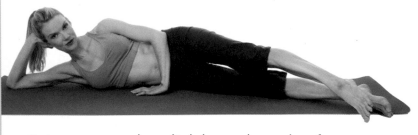

- Raise your top leg slightly, and tap that foot twice on the mat a few inches in front of your bottom foot.

- Lift your leg again, moving it to tap your top foot twice on the mat a few inches behind your bottom foot.

TONE	LOSS
Perform 4 reps in each direction on each leg	Perform 8 reps in each direction on each leg

- Lie on one side with your legs straight and stacked and your feet slightly apart. Prop up your head with one hand. Place your other hand on the mat in front of your stomach, bending your arm, for support.

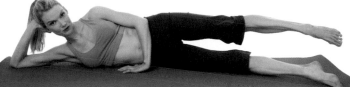

- Lift your top leg straight up, moving your top ankle directly over your hips and turning your foot out.

- Lower your leg, tapping your foot on the mat a few inches in front of your bottom foot.

- Raise the same leg high again, then lower it to tap the mat a few inches behind your bottom foot.

TONE	LOSS
Perform 4 reps in each direction on each leg	Perform 8 reps in each direction on each leg

#37 FLUTTER KICKS

- Lie on one side with your legs extended with feet together, slightly apart, and off the mat. Prop up your head with one hand. Place your other hand at the side of your head with your elbow pointed up and out.

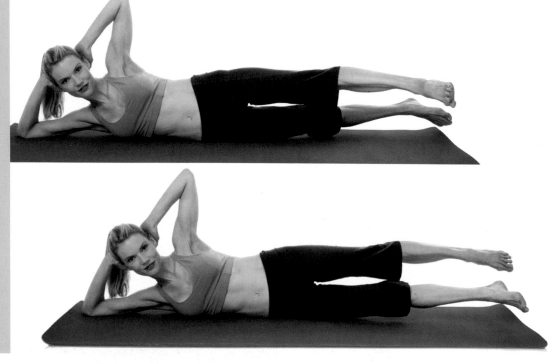

TONE	LOSS
Perform 8 reps back and forth on each side	Perform 16 reps back and forth on each side

- With both legs straight, kick your bottom leg forward as you move your top leg back.

- Quickly alternate your legs in a kicking motion.

- Lie on one side with your knees bent and your legs together in front. Prop up your head with one hand. Place your other hand on the mat in front of your stomach, bending your arm, for support.

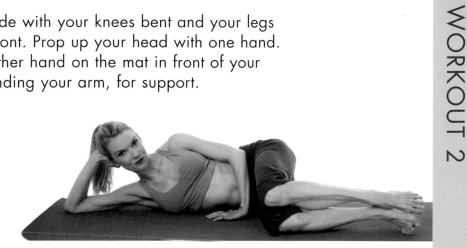

- Lift your top knee, moving from your hip to part your legs while keeping your feet touching and your bottom foot on the mat.

- Do not allow your pelvis to slide back as you lift your knee.

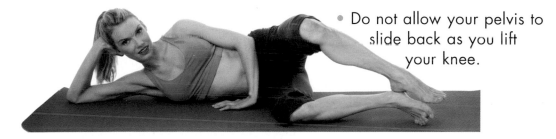

TONE	LOSS
Perform 4 reps on each side	Perform 8 reps on each side

#39 ADVANCED CLAM

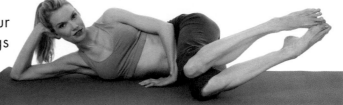

- Lie on one side with your knees bent and your legs together in front. Prop up your head with one hand. Place your other hand on the mat in front of your stomach, bending your arm, for support.

- Keep your bottom knee touching the mat as you lift your feet.

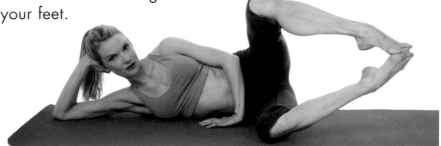

- Lift your top knee, moving from your hip to part your legs while keeping your feet touching in the air.

- Do not allow your pelvis to slide back as you lift your knee.

TONE	LOSS
Perform 4 reps on each side	Perform 8 reps on each side

- Lie face down on the mat with your legs extended straight behind you, your toes pointed, and the tops of your feet on the mat.

- Place your hands directly below your shoulders with your elbows pointing back.

- Slightly raise your head and shoulders off the mat.

- Push up your chest to a near straight-arm position, pulling your shoulders back and opening your chest. Look straight forward.

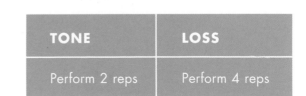

TONE	LOSS
Perform 2 reps	Perform 4 reps

#41 SWIMMING

- Lie face down on the mat with your legs extended straight behind you and your arms extended overhead.

- Lift one arm and your opposite leg about 18 inches off the mat.

- Slightly raise your head and upper torso.

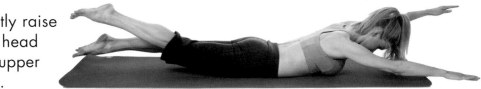

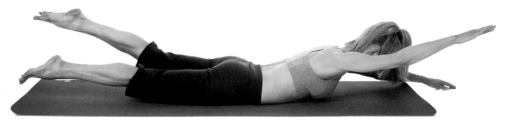

- Lower yourself slowly and repeat with your other arm and leg.

- Keep both your arms and legs straight and your head steady.

- You should feel the whole length of your spine as you perform the exercise.

TONE	LOSS
Perform 4 reps	Perform 8 reps

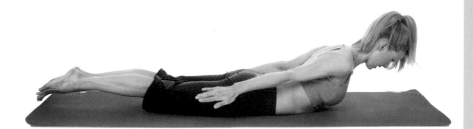

- Lie face down on the mat with your legs extended straight behind you and your arms extended overhead with your palms down.

- Lift your head, shoulders, and lower legs off the mat as you swing your arms into position at your sides, keeping your palms facing down.

- At the top position, only your thighs and stomach should touch the mat.

TONE	LOSS
Perform 2 reps	Perform 4 reps

#43 HEEL BEATS

- Lie face down on the mat, propped up on both forearms with your elbows under your shoulders and your legs extended straight behind you.

- Grip your right fist in your left hand.

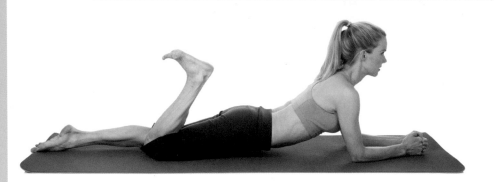

- Pick up one leg to kick your buttocks; pulse twice at the top.

- Lower the first leg as you raise the other leg and perform the kicks and pulses.

TONE	LOSS
Perform 4 reps of 2 beats on each leg	Perform 8 reps of 2 beats on each leg

#44 DOUBLE-HEEL BEATS

- Lie face down on the mat with your legs straight and your hands held together in the small of your back.

- Turn your head to one side and position it on the mat.

- Holding your legs together, move them toward your buttocks as if to kick them, pulsing at the top three times.

TONE	LOSS
Perform 4 reps of 2 beats	Perform 8 reps of 2 beats

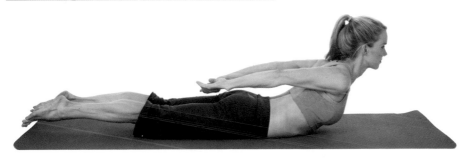

- Lower your legs toward the mat, keeping them a few inches above it.

- Stretch your arms back toward your feet and lift your head and shoulders.

- Return to the mat, placing your head on the other side, and repeat the exercise.

#45 FULL FOREARM PLANK

- Lie face down on the mat with your legs extended straight behind you and your arms tucked in at your sides with your elbows bent.

- Lift your body onto your toes and forearms, and hold the position briefly.

- Keep your back flat and your head slightly raised, looking forward.

TONE	LOSS
Hold for 30 seconds	Hold for 1 minute

- Lie face down on the mat with your legs extended straight behind you and your hands at your sides with your elbows bent.

- Touch your forehead to the mat.

- Push your upper body toward the ceiling to a straight-arm position, keeping your lower legs on the mat.

- Lower your upper body backward, bending your knees to rest on your haunches.

- Straighten your arms as you move back, but do not move your hands.

TONE	LOSS
Perform 2 reps	Perform 4 reps

#47 CHILD'S POSE

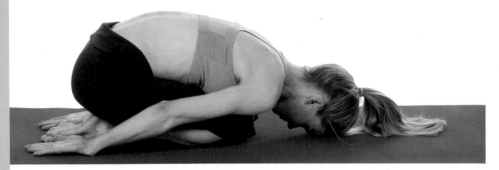

- Position yourself on all fours, then drop your hips down onto the backs of your legs.

- Lower your torso onto your upper thighs and your head to the mat. Move your arms into position along your sides with your palms up.

TONE	LOSS
Hold for 30 seconds	Hold for 1 minute

#1 CENTERING THE SPINE

- Lie on your back with your knees bent, your feet flat, and your arms straight by your sides with your palms down.

- Draw your navel toward your spine and inhale deeply as you center your spine.

- Exhale and repeat.

TONE	LOSS
Perform 3 reps	Perform 3 reps

#2 CERVICAL NOD AND CURL

- Lie on your back with your knees bent, your feet flat, and your arms straight by your sides with your palms down.

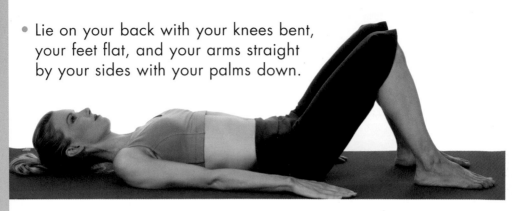

- Lift your head, shoulders, and hands off the mat, pulling your chin to your chest and drawing your navel toward your spine.

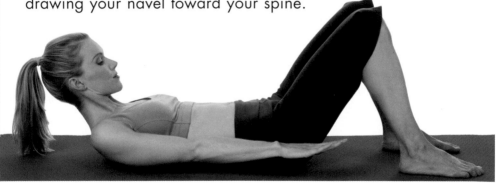

TONE	LOSS
Perform 3 reps	Perform 3 reps

- Lie on your back with your knees bent, your feet flat, and your arms straight by your sides with your palms down.

- Lift one foot off the mat about 12 inches, keeping the same bend at the knee.

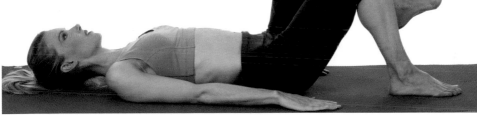

- Lower your foot and repeat with the other foot.

TONE	LOSS
Perform 4 reps on each leg	Perform 8 reps on each leg

#4 ARM CIRCLES

- Lie on your back with your knees bent, your feet flat, and your arms extended overhead with your palms up.

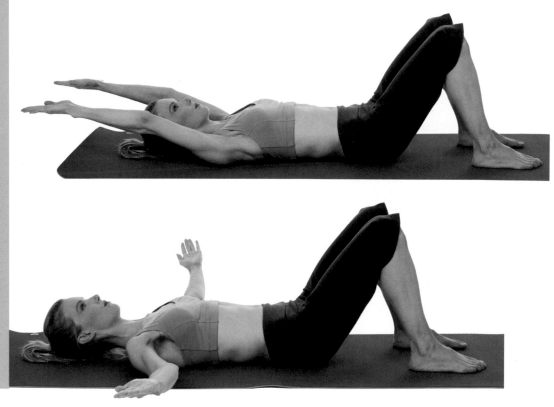

- Rotate your arms, moving them straight out to the sides and then down to your hips, coming together over your body's mid-line with your palms facing down.

- Repeat in the opposite direction.

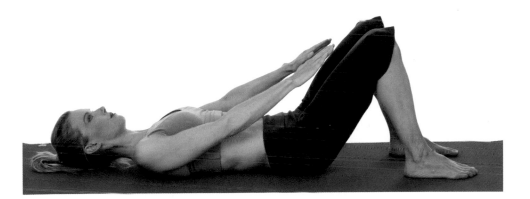

TONE	LOSS
Perform 3 reps in each direction	Perform 6 reps in each direction

#5 BUG

- Lie on your back with your knees bent and your feet lifted just above knee height at a 90-degree angle.

- Hold your arms straight up over your chest.

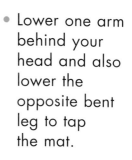

- Lower one arm behind your head and also lower the opposite bent leg to tap the mat.

- Lift both your arm and leg back to the mid-position, and repeat with the opposite arm and leg.

- Keep your knees bent throughout the exercise.

TONE	LOSS
Perform 4 reps to each side	Perform 8 reps to each side

#6 ADVANCED HUNDRED

- Lie on your back with your knees bent, your feet flat on the mat, and your arms straight by your sides with your palms down.

- Lift your head and shoulders off the mat, pulling your chin to your chest.

- Lift your legs up straight at a 45-degree angle.

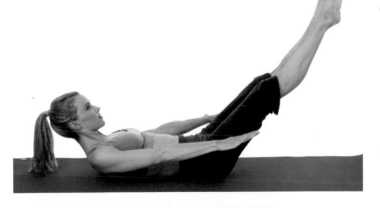

- Draw your navel toward your spine and pump your arms up and down about 12 inches as you breathe in.

- Repeat the pumping motion as you breathe out.

- Keep your head and shoulders up throughout the exercise.

TONE	LOSS
10 breaths with 5 arm pumps on inhale and 5 on exhale	10 breaths with 5 arm pumps on inhale and 5 on exhale

#7 SINGLE-LEG CIRCLES

- Lie on your back with your legs straight out and your arms straight by your sides with your palms down.

- Raise one leg straight up and turn that foot out slightly.

- Rotate your leg across your body, down and around, drawing a circle in the air with your foot.

- Reverse the movement, moving your leg in the opposite direction.

- Repeat with the other leg.

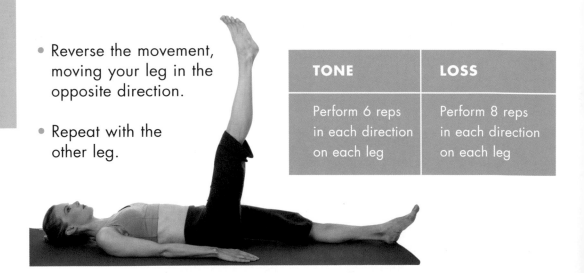

TONE	LOSS
Perform 6 reps in each direction on each leg	Perform 8 reps in each direction on each leg

- Lie on your back with your legs straight out and your arms extended overhead.

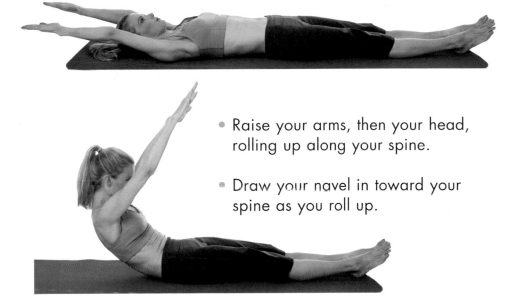

- Raise your arms, then your head, rolling up along your spine.

- Draw your navel in toward your spine as you roll up.

- Continue rolling forward, reaching past your feet. Do not touch your toes; stretch through your arms.

- Keep your shoulders relaxed and use your core muscles to perform the exercise.

- Reverse the movement as you roll back down.

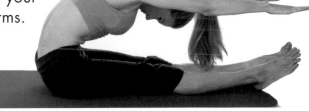

TONE	LOSS
Perform 4 reps	Perform 8 reps

#9 FORWARD SPINE STRETCH

- Sit upright with your legs straight out in front of you and your feet about hip-width apart.

- Extend your arms straight out in front at shoulder height with your palms down.

- Pull your chin toward your chest and draw your navel in toward your spine while reaching forward as if you were rounding yourself over a big ball.

- Reverse the movement, coming back to an upright seated position.

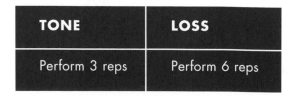

TONE	LOSS
Perform 3 reps	Perform 6 reps

#10 ROLL LIKE A BALL

- Sit upright with your knees bent, your feet flat, and your arms by your sides.

- Lift your feet slightly, bringing your heels toward your buttocks and gripping your ankles.

- Pull your chin in toward your chest and your navel toward your spine.

- Roll straight backward along your spine until your shoulders touch the mat.

- Roll back up to the starting position, keeping your feet lifted off the mat.

- Hold the same body position throughout the exercise.

TONE	LOSS
Perform 3 reps	Perform 6 reps

#11 SINGLE-LEG STRETCH

- Lie on your back with your legs extended and your arms straight by your sides with your palms down.

- Lift your head and shoulders off the mat, pulling your chin to your chest.

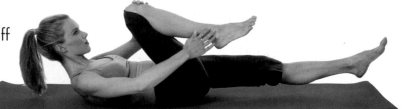

- Bring one knee into your chest, while slightly raising the other leg to a diagonal.

- Draw your navel toward your spine and draw the bent knee closer to your chest, placing one hand on your ankle and the other on your knee.

- Switch legs and hands, keeping your head stable and your back flat.

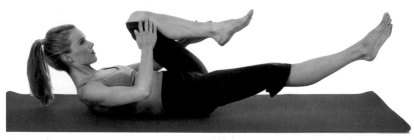

TONE	LOSS
Perform 8 reps on each leg	Perform 16 reps on each leg

#12 DOUBLE-LEG STRETCH

- Lie on your back with your knees bent and both feet lifted to knee height, forming a 90-degree angle.

- Lift your head and shoulders off the mat, pulling your chin to your chest and drawing your navel toward your spine.

- Position your hands at the sides of your shins.

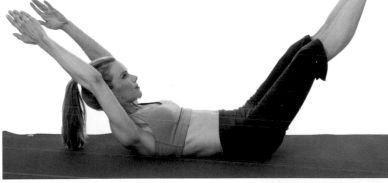

- Stretch your arms overhead close to your ears, and straighten your legs to a 45-degree angle.

- Return to the starting position, moving your arms out to your sides, and then back to your shins.

TONE	LOSS
Perform 8 reps of lowering and lifting	Perform 16 reps of lowering and lifting

#13 STRAIGHT-LEG SINGLE-LEG STRETCH

- Lie on your back with your legs extended on the mat, with your arms straight by your sides and your palms down.

- Keeping both legs straight, lift them about 12 inches off the mat.

- Lift your head and shoulders, pulling your chin to your chest.

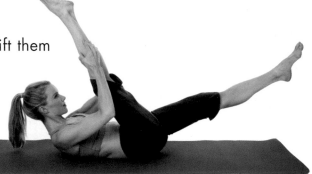

- Lift one leg straight up toward your head, gripping it with both hands behind your ankle or calf.

- Lower your leg and repeat with the other leg, keeping your arms, head, and shoulders up.

TONE	LOSS
Perform 8 reps on each leg	Perform 16 reps on each leg

#14 STRAIGHT-LEG DOUBLE-LEG STRETCH

- Lie on your back with your legs straight up and your hands at the sides of your head.

- Raise your head and shoulders off the mat, pulling your chin to your chest.

- Draw your navel toward your spine.

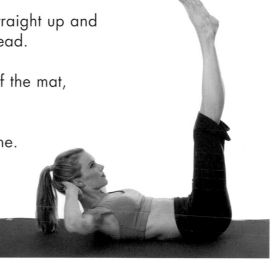

TONE	LOSS
Perform 8 reps of lowering and lifting	Perform 12 reps of lowering and lifting

- Lower your legs together about halfway down to the mat, and briefly hold the position, being sure to breathe.

- Return to the first position and repeat.

- Focus on using your core muscles to control the speed of your movement.

#15 CRISS CROSS

- Lie on your back with your knees bent and your feet raised to knee height.

- Place your hands at the sides of your head with your elbows wide apart.

- Lift your head and shoulders off the mat, pulling your chin to your chest.

- Extend one leg at a 45-degree angle, then twist your torso to the opposite side, bringing your elbow toward the opposite bent knee.

- Switch sides and legs, keeping your elbows wide apart.

TONE	LOSS
Perform 8 reps to each side	Perform 16 reps to each side

- Sit upright with your legs straight out in front and your feet shoulder-width apart.

- Lift your arms straight up and hold them out to the sides at shoulder height. Draw your navel toward your spine.

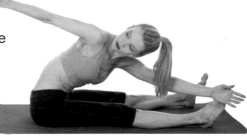

- Bending from your hips, twist your torso down to one side and extend your hand to the outside of the opposite ankle.

- Stretch the other arm back while turning your head to look back.

- Pulse three times toward your foot, as if your pinky finger were sawing off your little toe.

- Return to the upright seated position and repeat on the other side.

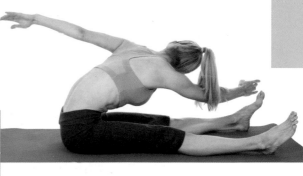

TONE	LOSS
Perform 2 reps to each side with 3 pulses	Perform 4 reps to each side with 3 pulses

#17 ADVANCED OPEN-LEG ROCKER

- Sit with your knees bent, your feet flat, and your hands on your ankles. Draw your navel in toward your spine.

- Sit back on your buttocks and lift your feet off the mat, bringing them up to knee height.

- Straightening your legs, hold them at a 45-degree angle.

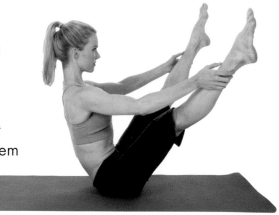

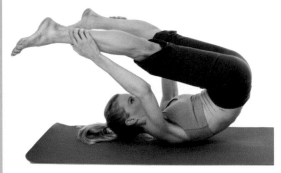

- With your feet about shoulder-width apart, roll back to the tops of your shoulders.

- Roll back to the upright position.

- Keep your legs straight and your feet apart throughout the exercise.

TONE	LOSS
Perform 3 reps	Perform 6 reps

#18 ROLL OVER

- Lie on your back with your legs straight up and your arms straight by your sides with your palms down.

- With your feet hip-width apart, lift your legs back over your head.

- When your legs are parallel to the mat, close your feet and slowly roll back down.

- Open your legs until they are again hip-width apart and repeat for the required reps.

- Repeat the entire sequence, this time starting with your legs closed and then opening them overhead.

TONE	LOSS
Perform 1 rep with feet open, then 1 rep with feet together	Perform 3 reps with feet open, then 3 reps with feet together

#19 TICK TOCK

- Lie on your back with your legs straight up and with your ankles directly over your hips.

- Position your arms straight out to your sides at shoulder height.

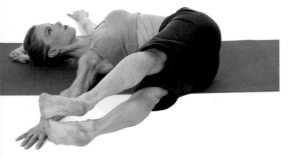

- With your legs together, roll your hips to one side, almost touching your outside foot to the mat.

- Using your core muscles, lift your legs back to the mid-position.

- Roll your hips to the opposite side, again almost touching your foot to the mat.

- Keep your legs straight and your upper body stable throughout.

TONE	LOSS
Perform 8 reps to each side	Perform 12 reps to each side

#20 TICK TOCK WITH WALKING

- Lie on your back with your legs straight up and your arms straight out at your sides at shoulder height.

- Roll your legs to one side, almost touching your foot to the mat.

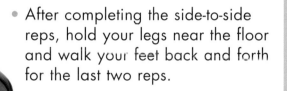

- After completing the side-to-side reps, hold your legs near the floor and walk your feet back and forth for the last two reps.

- Lift your legs back to the center and repeat on the other side.

TONE	LOSS
Perform 4 reps with each foot, walking your feet 4 steps for the last two reps	Perform 8 reps with each foot, walking your feet 8 steps for the last two reps

#21 ADVANCED CORKSCREW

- Lie on your back with your legs straight up at a 45-degree angle.

- Place your hands by your sides with your palms down.

- Turn your feet out into the Pilates stance, keeping your heels touching.

- Roll back to lower your legs behind your head, rolling onto your shoulders.

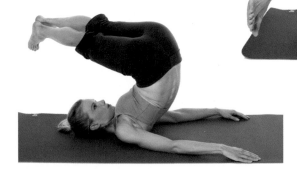

- Using your core muscles, rotate your legs around your head and down at a 45-degree angle, drawing a big circle in the air.

- Reverse the direction of your rotation.

TONE	LOSS
Perform 2 reps in each direction	Perform 4 reps in each direction

#22 EXTENDED-LEG HIP BRIDGE

- Lie on your back with your knees bent, your feet flat, and your arms straight by your sides with your palms down.

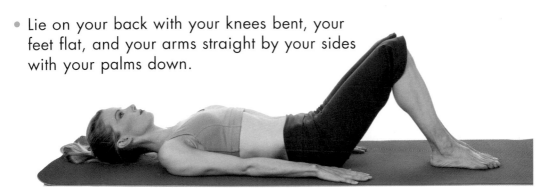

- Lift your hips off the mat, forming a straight line from your knees to your shoulders.

- Extend one leg straight out and point your foot.

- Lower yourself back to the mat and repeat the exercise with your other leg.

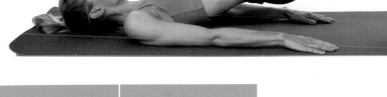

TONE	LOSS
Perform 4 reps on each leg	Perform 8 reps on each leg

#23 HIP BRIDGE THRUST

- Lie on your back with your knees bent, your feet flat, and your arms straight by your sides with your palms down.

- Raise one leg straight up, flexing your foot.

- Lift your hips off the mat, forming a straight line from your bent knee to your shoulders.

- Lower yourself back to the mat and perform the required number of reps.

- Switch sides and repeat the exercise with the other leg.

TONE	LOSS
Perform 4 reps on each leg	Perform 8 reps on each leg

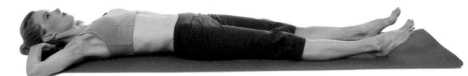

- Lie on your back with your legs extended and your feet hip-width apart.

- Position your hands at the sides of your head with your elbows out to the sides.

- Carefully roll up off the mat, pulling your navel in toward your spine.

- Continue rolling forward toward your feet, lowering your head to your knees.

- Sit up straight and start to lean back at an angle, then reverse the movement, rolling back to the starting position.

- Keep your elbows wide throughout the exercise.

TONE	LOSS
Perform 2 reps	Perform 4 reps

#25 NECK PULL TWIST

- Sit upright with your back flat and your hands positioned behind your head with your elbows open and pointed out.

- Lean back to a 45-degree angle, then twist your head and shoulders to one side.

- Sit up straight and repeat, twisting to the opposite side.

- Do not allow your hips to shift; twist from your waist, keeping your abdomen pulled in.

- Keep your elbows opened wide throughout the exercise.

TONE	LOSS
Perform 2 reps to each side	Perform 4 reps to each side

#26 SHAVING

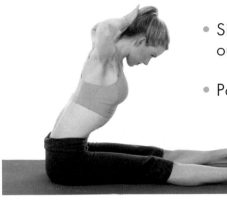

- Sit upright with your legs extended straight out in front and your feet hip-width apart.

- Position your hands behind your head with your elbows out to the sides. Lean slightly forward from your hips and hold your thumb and index fingers together.

- Straighten your arms overhead at a 45-degree angle, as if you were shaving the back of your neck.

- Move your hands back behind your head and repeat the exercise.

- Keep your back flat throughout the exercise and be sure your palms face your head. Relax your shoulders as you stretch your arms out and back.

TONE	LOSS
Perform 8 reps	Perform 16 reps

#27 TWIST

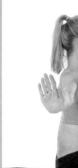

- Sit upright with your legs extended straight out in front and your feet shoulder-width apart.

- Lift your arms straight up and out to the sides at shoulder height with your hands pointing up.

- Draw your navel toward your spine and twist from your waist 90 degrees to one side.

- Twist back to the middle, and then to the opposite side.

- Keep your arms up at shoulder height and your fingers pointing up throughout the exercise.

TONE	LOSS
Perform 2 reps to each side	Perform 4 reps to each side

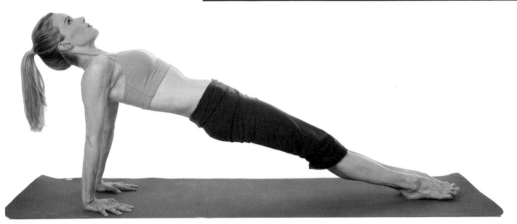

- Sit on the mat with your legs extended straight out in front.

- Position your hands about 12 inches behind your buttocks with your palms down.

- Lift your hips off the mat, keeping your legs straight and your feet pointed.

- Come up into a straight-arm position and hold it briefly.

- Keep your head up and look toward the ceiling.

TONE	LOSS
Hold for 30 seconds	Hold for 1 minute

#29 LEG PULL UP

- Start in the Incline Plank position (page 127) with your arms and legs extended straight and your toes pointed.

- Draw your navel toward your spine and lift one leg straight up as high as you can.

- Pulse twice at the top.

TONE	LOSS
Perform 2 reps on each leg	Perform 4 reps on each leg

- Lower your leg, and repeat with your other leg.

- Keep your arms and legs straight throughout the exercise.

#30 TRICEPS DIP

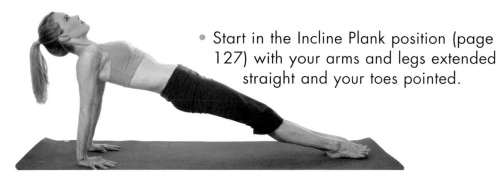

- Start in the Incline Plank position (page 127) with your arms and legs extended straight and your toes pointed.

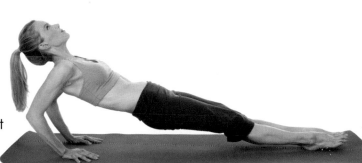

- Bend your elbows, lowering your body toward the floor.

- Keep your legs straight and feet pointed.

- Press up to a straight-arm position; keep your head up and look toward the ceiling.

TONE	LOSS
Perform 4 reps	Perform 8 reps

#31 SINGLE-LEG TEASER

- Lie flat on your back with your knees bent, your feet flat, and your arms extended overhead.

- Lift one leg straight up to a 70-degree angle.

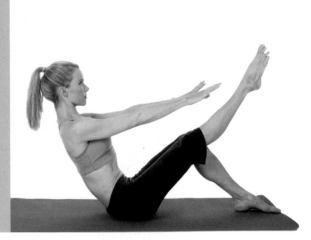

- Lift your arms, then your head and shoulders to roll up.

- Continue rolling up into a V-shape, reaching toward the toes of your raised leg.

- Lengthen through the sides of your waist, keeping your knees pressed together.

- Roll back down to the mat.

TONE	LOSS
Perform 2 reps on each leg	Perform 4 reps on each leg

#32 SINGLE-LEG TEASER WITH TWIST

- Lie flat on your back with your knees bent, your feet flat, and your arms extended overhead.

- Lift one leg straight up to a 70-degree angle.

- Lift your arms, then your head and shoulders, to roll up.

- Continue rolling up into a V-shape, reaching toward the toes of your raised leg.

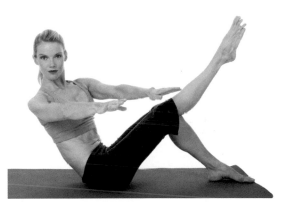

- Twist your torso, shoulders, and head to the straight-leg side.

- Lengthen through the sides of your waist, keeping your knees pressed together.

- Straighten your torso and roll back down to the mat.

TONE	LOSS
Perform 2 reps on each leg	Perform 4 reps on each leg

#33 ADVANCED TEASER

- Lie flat on your back with your arms extended overhead and your legs extended straight.

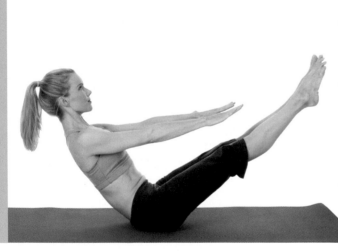

- Lift your legs to a 45-degree angle.

- Raise your arms, then your head and shoulders, rolling your upper body up off the mat.

- Continue rolling up into a V-shape, reaching toward your toes.

- Lower your upper body back to the mat.

TONE	LOSS
Perform 2 reps	Perform 4 reps

#34 ADVANCED TEASER WITH TWIST

- Lie flat on your back with your arms extended overhead and your legs straight out in front.

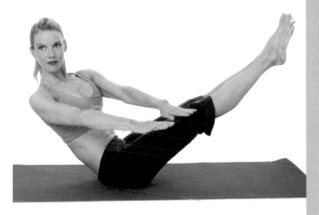

- Raise your legs to a 45-degree angle.

- Raise your arms, then your head and shoulders, rolling your upper body off the mat.

- Continue rolling up into a V-shape, reaching toward your toes.

- Twist your torso, shoulders, and head to one side.

- Straighten your torso and roll back down to the mat.

- Repeat the twist to the other side.

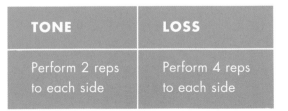

TONE	LOSS
Perform 2 reps to each side	Perform 4 reps to each side

#35 STIRRING BUBBLES

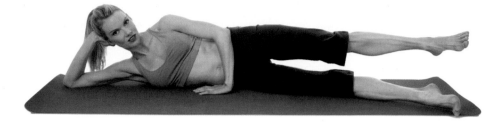

- Lie on one side with your legs straight out. Prop up your head with one hand. Place the other hand on the mat in front of your stomach, bending your arm, for support.

- Turn your top leg out from the hip socket and point your toes.

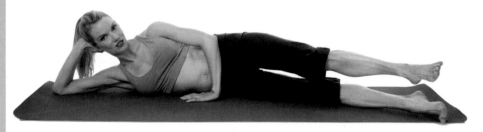

- Rotate your top leg forward, making small circles in the air.

- Reverse the movement, making small circles in the opposite direction.

TONE	LOSS
Perform 8 circles forward, then 8 backward, on each side	Perform 12 circles forward, then 12 backward, on each side

- Lie on one side with your legs straight and slightly in front. Prop up your head with one hand. Place the other hand on the mat in front of your stomach, bending your arm, for support.

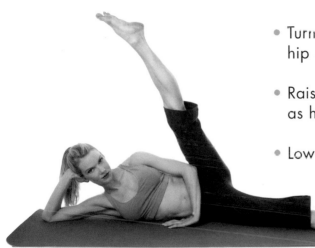

- Turn your top leg out from the hip socket.

- Raise your top leg up straight, as high as you can.

- Lower your leg and repeat.

TONE	LOSS
Perform 4 reps on each leg	Perform 8 reps on each leg

#37 PASSÉ

- Lie on one side with your legs straight and slightly in front of your body. Prop up your head with one hand. Place your other hand on the mat in front of your stomach, bending your arm, for support.

- Raise your top leg up straight, as high as you can.

- Bend your top knee and lower your foot to touch your bottom knee, then straighten the leg again.

- Lower your leg back to the starting position. Repeat the entire sequence, this time bending your knee first and then straightening your leg toward the ceiling.

TONE	LOSS
Perform 4 reps on each leg	Perform 8 reps on each leg

#38 FORWARD AND BACK KICKS

- Lie on one side with your legs out straight and slightly in front of your body. Prop your head up with one hand. Place the other hand on the mat in front of your stomach, bending your arm, for support.

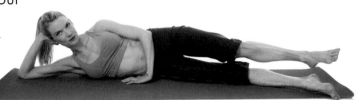

- Draw your navel toward your spine and kick your top leg forward from the hip, pulsing once at the front position.

- Swing your leg back behind and then forward again.

- Keep your hips stacked one on top of the other and keep your feet flexed with your toes pointed.

TONE	LOSS
Perform 4 reps on each leg	Perform 8 reps on each leg

WORKOUT 3

#39 BICYCLE

- Lie on one side with your legs out straight and slightly in front of your body. Prop your head up with one hand. Place your other hand on the mat in front of your stomach, bending your arm, for support.

- Draw your navel in toward your spine and kick your top leg straight forward from the hip.

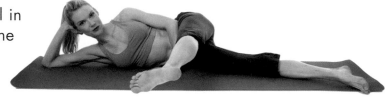

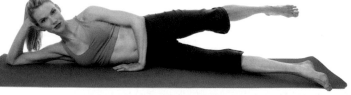

- Bend your top knee and draw your top leg back behind you.

- Straighten your top leg behind, then swing it forward to repeat the pedaling motion.

- Stop and reverse the direction, bending your knee as you come forward and straightening your leg when it's in front.

- Swing your leg back straight and then repeat the exercise.

TONE	LOSS
Perform 4 reps on each leg	Perform 8 reps on each leg

- Lie on one side with your legs straight and stacked. Prop up

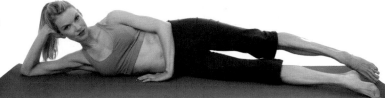

your head with one hand. Place your other hand on the mat in front of your stomach, bending your arm, for support.

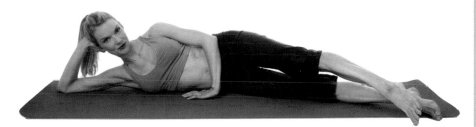

- Raise your top leg slightly, and tap that foot twice on the mat a few inches in front of your bottom foot.

- Lift your leg again, moving your foot to tap twice on the mat a few inches behind your bottom foot.

TONE	LOSS
Perform 8 reps in each direction on each leg	Perform 16 reps in each direction on each leg

#41 AROUND THE WORLD

- Lie on one side with your legs straight and stacked and your feet slightly apart. Prop up your head with one hand. Place your other hand on the mat in front of your stomach, bending your arm, for support.

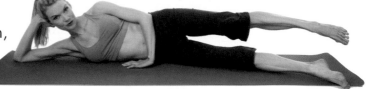

- Lift your top leg straight up, moving your top ankle directly over your hips and turning your foot out.

- Lower your leg, tapping your foot on the mat a few inches in front of your bottom foot.

- Raise the same leg high again, then lower it to tap the mat a few inches behind your bottom foot.

TONE	LOSS
Perform 4 reps in each direction on each leg	Perform 8 reps in each direction on each leg

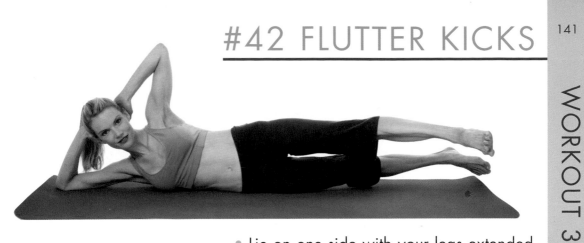

- Lie on one side with your legs extended and your feet together, slightly apart and off the mat. Prop up your head with one hand. Place your other hand at the side of your head with your elbow pointing up.

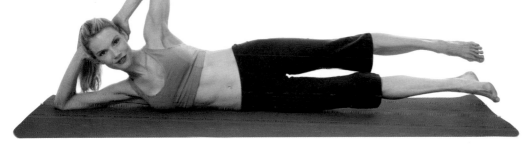

- With both legs straight, kick your bottom leg forward as you move your top leg back.

- Quickly alternate your legs in a kicking motion.

TONE	LOSS
Perform 8 reps back and forth on each side	Perform 16 reps back and forth on each side

#43 SIDE PLANK WITH TWIST

WORKOUT 3

- Lie on your side with your legs straight and stacked on top of each other and your bottom arm bent with your elbow directly under your shoulder.

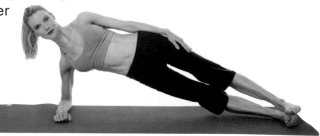

- Lift your body off the mat, resting on your forearm and foot.

- Keep the other arm straight along your side.

- Raise your top arm straight toward the ceiling.

TONE	LOSS
Perform 2 reps on each side, holding for 4 breaths each time	Perform 4 reps on each side, holding for 4 breaths each time

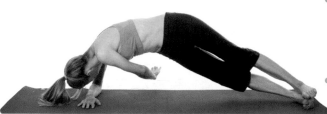

- Lower your top arm down and around, twisting to reach under your chest.

- Return to the top position.

- Lie on one side with your knees bent and your legs extended together in front of you. Prop up your head with one hand. Place your other hand on the mat in front of your stomach, bending your arm, for support.

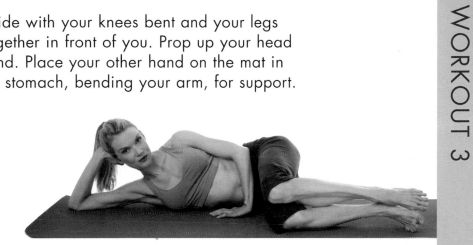

- Lift your top knee, moving from your hip to part your legs while keeping your feet touching and your bottom foot on the mat.

- Do not allow your pelvis to slide back as you lift your knee.

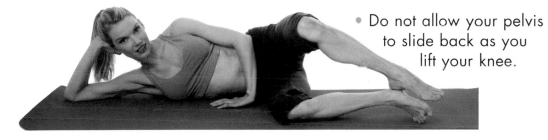

TONE	LOSS
Perform 4 reps on each side	Perform 8 reps on each side

#45 ADVANCED CLAM

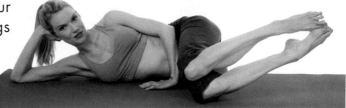

- Lie on one side with your knees bent and your legs together out in front. Prop up your head with one hand. Place your other hand on the mat in front of your stomach, bending your arm, for support.

- Keep your bottom knee touching the mat as you lift your feet.

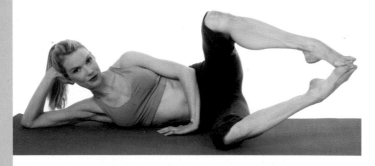

- Lift your top knee, moving from your hip to part your legs while keeping your feet touching in the air.

- Do not allow your pelvis to slide back as you lift your knee.

TONE	LOSS
Perform 4 reps on each side	Perform 8 reps on each side

- Lie on one side with your knees bent and legs together out in front. Prop up your head with one hand. Place your other hand on the mat in front of your stomach, bending your arm, for support.

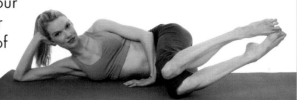

- Keep your bottom knee touching the mat as you lift your feet.

- Lift your top knee, moving from your hip to part your legs, while keeping your feet touching in the air.

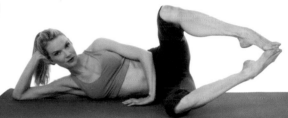

- Kick your top leg out at a 45-degree angle.

- Bend your top leg back in, then close your legs again.

- Do not allow your pelvis to slide back as you lift your leg.

TONE	LOSS
Perform 4 reps on each side	Perform 8 reps on each side

#47 COBRA

- Lie face down on the mat with your legs extended straight behind you, your toes pointed, and the tops of your feet on the mat.

- Place your hands directly below your shoulders with your elbows pointing back.

- Slightly raise your head and shoulders off the mat.

- Push up your chest to a near straight-arm position, pulling your shoulders back and opening your chest. Look straight forward.

TONE	LOSS
Perform 2 reps	Perform 4 reps

#48 SWIMMING

- Lie face down on the mat with your legs extended straight behind you and your arms extended overhead with your palms down.
- Lift one arm and your opposite leg about 18 inches off the mat. Slightly raise your head and upper torso.

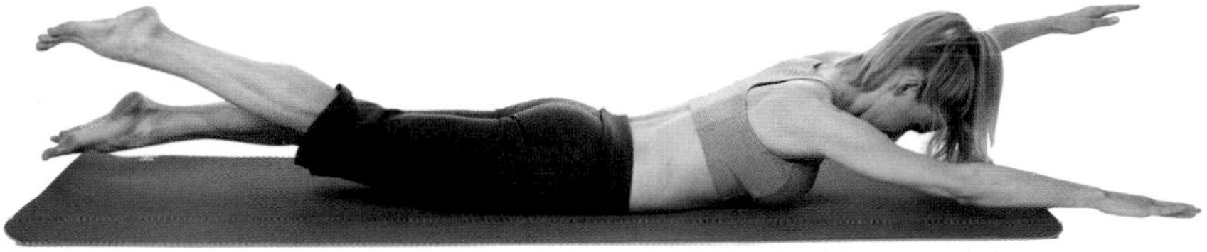

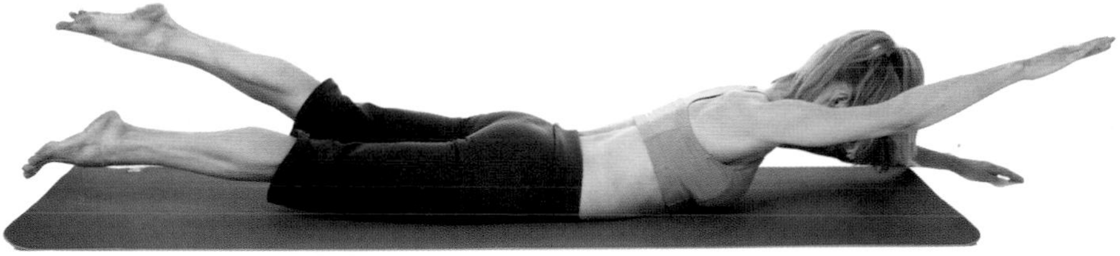

- Lower yourself slowly and repeat with your other arm and leg.
- Keep both your arms and legs straight and your head steady.
- You should feel the whole length of your spine as you perform the exercise.

TONE	LOSS
Perform 8 reps	Perform 16 reps

#49 SWAN

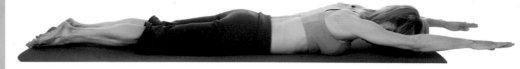

- Lie face down on the mat with your legs extended straight behind you and your arms extended overhead with your palms down.

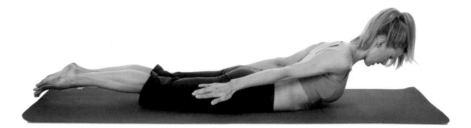

- Lift your head, shoulders, and lower legs off the mat as you swing your arms into position at your sides, keeping your palms facing down.

- At the top position, only your thighs and stomach should touch the mat.

TONE	LOSS
Perform 2 reps	Perform 4 reps

#50 SWAN DIVE

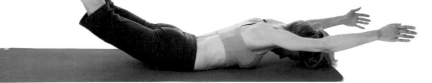

- Lie face down on the mat with your head and shoulders up and your arms straight out in front.

- Lift your hands, swinging your arms up in front.

- Dive forward, rolling up your chest as you swing your legs up behind you.

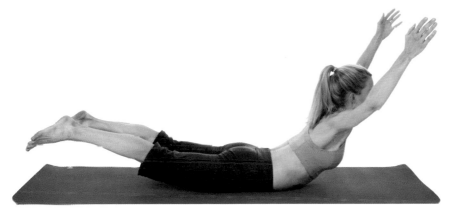

- Use the momentum of the forward roll to swing back, pitching your upper body up in the air again.

TONE	LOSS
Perform 2 reps	Perform 4 reps

#51 HEEL BEATS

- Lie face down on the mat, propped up on both forearms with your elbows under your shoulders and your legs extended straight behind you.

- Grip your right fist in your left hand.

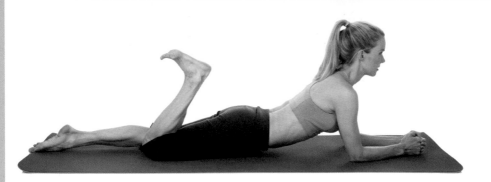

- Pick up one leg to kick your buttocks; pulse twice at the top.

- Lower the first leg as you raise the other leg and perform the kicks and pulses.

TONE	LOSS
Perform 4 reps of 2 beats on each leg	Perform 8 reps of 2 beats on each leg

#52 DOUBLE-HEEL BEATS

- Lie face down on the mat with your legs straight and your hands held together in the small of your back.

- Turn your head to one side and position it on the mat.

- Holding your legs together, move them toward your buttocks, as if to kick them, pulsing at the top three times.

- Lower your legs toward the mat, keeping them a few inches above it.

- Stretch your arms back toward your feet and lift your head and shoulders.

- Return to the mat, placing your head on the other side, and repeat the exercise.

TONE	LOSS
Perform 4 reps of 2 beats	Perform 8 reps of 2 beats

#53 FULL FOREARM PLANK

- Lie face down on the mat with your legs extended straight behind you and your arms tucked in at your sides with your elbows bent.

- Lift your body onto your toes and forearms, and hold the position briefly.

- Keep your back flat and your head slightly raised, looking forward.

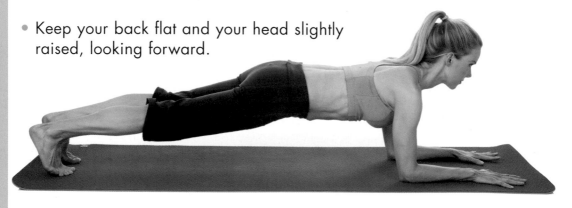

TONE	LOSS
Hold for 30 seconds	Hold for 1 minute

#54 LITTLE PIECE OF HEAVEN

- Lie face down on the mat with your legs straight behind you and your hands at your sides with your elbows bent.

- Touch your forehead to the mat.

- Push your upper body toward the ceiling to a straight-arm position, keeping your lower legs on the mat.

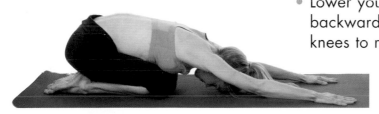

- Lower your upper body backward, bending your knees to rest on your haunches.

- Straighten your arms as you move back, but do not move your hands.

TONE	LOSS
Perform 2 reps	Perform 4 reps

#55 CHILD'S POSE

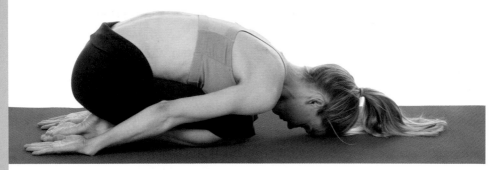

- Position yourself on all fours, then drop your hips down onto the backs of your legs.

- Lower your torso onto your upper thighs and your head to the mat. Move your arms into position along your sides with your palms up.

TONE	LOSS
Hold for 30 seconds	Hold for 1 minute

#56 PILATES PUSH-UP TO WALK OUT TO WALK BACK

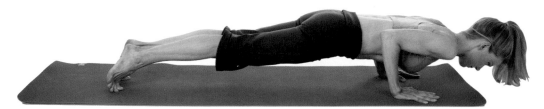

PILATES PUSH-UP

- Start in a plank position, or at the bottom of a push-up, with your body lifted straight off the mat, as you rest on your toes and hands with your elbows bent.

- Push up to a straight-arm position.

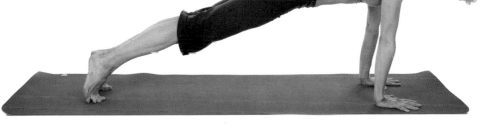

- Lower yourself back to the plank position, keeping your elbows tucked in against your ribs.

- Push up again, and walk your hands in to your feet.

WALK OUT

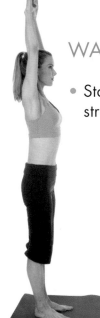

- Stand upright with your arms stretched overhead.

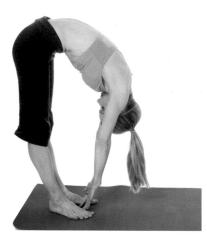

- Roll forward one vertebra at a time, lifting your abdominals and lowering your hands to the mat.

- Walk your hands out in front, keeping your legs straight.

- Move into a straight-body position, finishing at the top of a push-up.

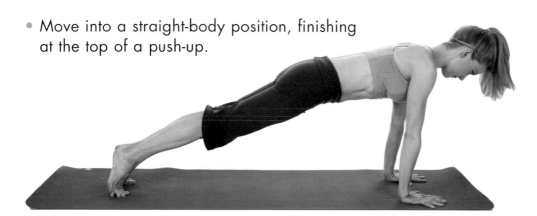

- Lower your body to the floor, bending your elbows.

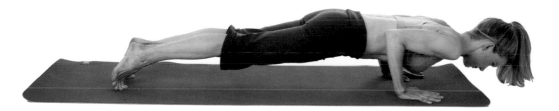

WALK BACK

- From the top of a push-up, walk your hands back under your body as you raise your hips.

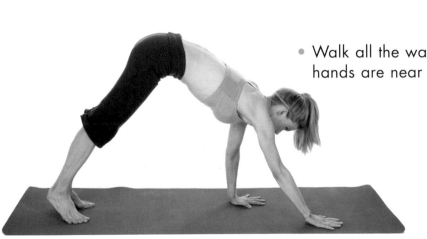

- Walk all the way in until your hands are near your feet.

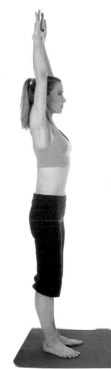

- Lift and straighten your upper body to come to a full upright position. Stretch your arms overhead.

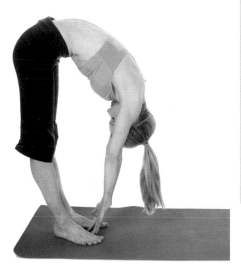

- Keep your legs straight throughout the exercise.

- Repeat the sequence of movements, starting from the Pilates Push-Up to the Walk Out and finishing with the Walk Back.

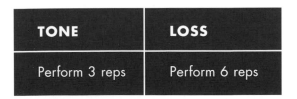

TONE	LOSS
Perform 3 reps	Perform 6 reps

INDEX